The period of adolescence and young adulthood is important as a time during which young people come to make sense of the society in which they live, and is a period in which their aspirations for the future become consolidated. This book deals with a specific group: deaf young people, as their deafness will have implications for their communication within both the family and society in general, with consequences for the way in which they come to understand the world.

This is a longitudinal follow up to the study reported in *The Deaf Child and his Family*, now re-published as *Deaf Children and their Families*. Some 18 years on, 75% of the original families have been traced and this new volume provides an account of the subsequent interviews with both the parents and the deaf young people themselves. Participants reflect not only on the consequences of deafness within their own lives, but also on the changing context for deaf people. It includes a comparison of the views of parents with those of their sons and daughters, and an examination of factors in early life that may relate to later development.

In its provision of a unique insight into the deaf young person's perspective on life, it will be a valuable resource for all those concerned with deafness and special education, including deaf people themselves, families, professionals and academics.

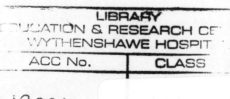

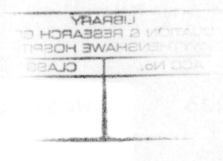

Deaf Young People and their Families: Developing Understanding

Deaf Young People and their Families:

Developing Understanding

SUSAN GREGORY
Senior Lecturer in Psychology, The Open University

JULIET BISHOP
Senior Counsellor, The Open University

and

LESLEY SHELDON
Specialist Social Worker (Child Protection),
Scunthorpe and Goole Hospital Trust

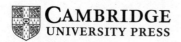
CAMBRIDGE
UNIVERSITY PRESS

Published by the Press Syndicate of the University of Cambridge
The Pitt Building, Trumpington Street, Cambridge CB2 1RP
40 West 20th Street, New York NY 10011-4211, USA
10 Stamford Road, Oakleigh, Melbourne 3166, Australia

First published 1995

Printed in Great Britain at the University Press, Cambridge

A catalogue record for this book is avaialable from the British Library

Library of Congress cataloguing in publication data available

ISBN 0 521 41977 8 hardback
ISBN 0 521 42998 6 paperback

SE

CONTENTS

PREFACE

This book is about deaf young people and their families. It is a follow up to the study reported in *The Deaf Child and his Family* (George Allen and Unwin, 1976) republished as *Deaf Children and their Families* to coincide with the publication of this book. In the first study, 122 families of young deaf children were interviewed. The authors of the present book set out some 18 years later to trace as many of a sample of 101 of the original families as possible, and established contact with 91 of them. This book is an account of the interviews with both the parents and the deaf young people themselves, and also includes comparative information from the earlier research and material from group discussions conducted with some of the young people who were interviewed.

The purpose of this book is to give the perspective of the young people and families themselves rather than a professional view. The period from the first interviews to the second set was a time of great change in the understanding of deafness and in professional approaches to it. This book allows participants to reflect not only on the consequences of deafness within their own lives, but also on the changing context for deaf people. It also allows a consideration of the similarities and dissimilarities in the views of parents and their sons and daughters on various issues and an examination of factors in early life that may relate to later development.

Notes on the transcription of quotes

All quotes have been taken from interviews or discussions that have taken place in connection with the research,

(a) with parents when the deaf young people were six years old or less (Parents C),

(b)   with parents of the young deaf people (Parents YP),
(c)   with the young deaf people themselves, and
(d)   with some of the young deaf people in group discussions.

Quotes are designated by a pseudonym for the deaf young person which is the same in all publications of the research. For Parents (C) interviews, the age of the child at the time of interview is given together with the page number for the quote in *Deaf Children and their Families* (DCF) if it is included there.

For interviews with the young people, and with the parents of the young people, the preferred language of the deaf young person is given together with the age at the time of the parent interview. Occasionally such information is omitted to protect confidentiality.

Hesitations and pauses in the quotes are indicated by dots...Omissions are indicated by parentheses () and supplementary information to clarify is provided in parentheses. A letter plus dots (A...) indicates the omission of a name to protect confidentiality.

ACKNOWLEDGEMENTS

This research has benefited greatly from conversations, discussions and debates with many people, both those directly involved in the project and other colleagues and friends.

Firstly, we would like to thank our note-takers, who assisted at the interviews with the young people. Not only were they concerned to ensure we had the fairest and fullest possible account of each interview, but their insights into the interview process and the issues we were addressing were very important to us. They were: Sue Barlow, Karen Beggs, Frances Connor, Martin Farrelly, Isabel Gregory, Karen Hale, Brenda Kent, Mike Poulton, Janice Silo, Steve Silo and Audrey Smith.

We would like to thank our friends and colleagues for interesting and constructive discussions which not only stimulated and clarified our thinking, but also encouraged us in planning and developing the research: Doug Alker, Sarah Beazley, Mairian Corker, Ann Darby, Karen Gowing, Gillian Hartley, Carlo Laurenzi, Clive Mason, Michele Moore, John Newson, Elizabeth Newson, Gloria Pullen, Alison Read, Sandra Smith, George Taylor, Alison Wells. The responsibility for the opinions and ideas expressed in the book, however, remains ours.

In particular, we would like to acknowledge the help we received from Jeanette Lilley on computer and statistical matters and Rukhsana Meherali on issues related to minority ethnic groups. We are grateful for the secretarial support we have received from Yvonne Holmes, who not only typed interview schedules, transcribed interviews and prepared drafts of the book, but assisted with contacting interviewees, answering queries and other administrative tasks. We would also like to thank Lin Clark and Julia Montague, who helped with transcribing and typing interviews. We are also grateful to Rosemary Hurdman for allowing Lesley to modify her contract in order that she could work on the research.

We appreciate the support of our families throughout the period of the study – our partners, Keir, David and Mike; and our sons and daughters, the four who were with us throughout: Tilly, Isabel, Lizzy and Iven, and the four who joined us while the research was in progress, Ben, Abigail, Joanna and Isabella.

The main study reported here was funded by a grant from the Leverhulme Trust; the earlier research was funded by the National Deaf Children's Society. The research was also facilitated by grants from The Open University to allow participation in conferences, and study leave to enable the book to be written. We are extremely grateful to all these organisations for their financial support and also their encouragement.

The book is dedicated, however, to those without whom it would not have been possible, the parents and the young people themselves.

CHAPTER ONE

The young deaf people and their families

I want hearing people to learn about deaf people
Isabel

In your wildest dreams you cannot imagine the way I feel
Isabel's mother

Isabel is an articulate young deaf person. She has a good command of English, though not everyone could understand her speech. She uses English with her parents and hearing friends, and sign language with her deaf friends. In an interview, she described how she signed in her dreams and explained 'It's something to do with having a signing mind'. When she was young she thought that when she grew up she would be hearing as all the adults she knew could hear. She and her deaf friends used to discuss this at school, looking forward to the time when they would talk as quickly and easily as their parents did. However, by the time she was seven or eight years old, she realised she would always be deaf. She was always educated alongside other deaf pupils but she felt it was worse for her deaf boyfriend who went to a school with all hearing pupils, as he was very lonely and thought he was 'the only deaf person in the world.'

As an adult, Isabel explained 'I am happy to be deaf', though she also added that if there was an operation that was successful in restoring hearing she would consider it. She described her relationship with her boyfriend as 'beautiful' as they cared for and helped each other. She felt it would be difficult with a hearing boyfriend because, although when they were alone together they could probably communicate easily, in a group of hearing people she would find it difficult to follow the conversation and that could lead to problems. She said:

I once had a hearing boyfriend, and if we were out and I couldn't understand he'd say 'I'll explain later'. Then when we got home I'd ask but he could never remember. That upset me. I've been through all of that. It was a terrible time, I was really hurt.

At the time of the interviews, Isabel was working as a personal assistant in a large company, a post which required only a good general educational background and which offered no further training. She would have preferred to be a teacher and hoped to go to college at some time in the future to train for a position that would be more demanding. She said she was happy at work and found the job interesting, particularly when she detected errors in the bills that were sent in. Her mother was not so sure.

I don't think Isabel's talents have been fully tapped, but I think it's the deafness again. () She thinks it is totally boring what she is doing, but she realises the money is good and that she is lucky to have a job because she is disabled. This is not the way I feel, but how she feels. She hears of so many friends of hers that are out of work because nobody really wants to know them. () With Isabel being deaf, promotion is not easy. () There are not many jobs you can do without using the telephone.

Isabel was two months old when her parents first noticed that she did not seem to respond to sound, although it was not until she was two years old that the doctor finally confirmed she was deaf. Her mother reported that the doctor said:

'Mrs A... you've definitely got a problem. Isabel is deaf.' That was all. That was all I was told at the clinic, and I was very upset.

Isabel was a lively, alert child who was rarely miserable. She enjoyed drawing, writing, her climbing frame and her swing. In an interview when Isabel was nearly four years old, her mother said she enjoyed Isabel because 'she's her' and said she would not swap her for anything. Decisions that had to be made about Isabel's education were difficult. Should she go to the local school, or a specialist school for deaf children some distance away? Should sign language be used in her education, or should it be strictly speech- and English-based? Ultimately she went to a specialist boarding school, which used a spoken language approach, at 11 years of age.

In a second interview with this mother, when Isabel was 21 years old, she said:

I could never see the light at the end of the tunnel. I think that what it is, I could never see Isabel developing into the person she is today. () I felt she would be always and for ever needing help which she doesn't.

In both these interviews Isabel's mother talked of the lack of information about deafness, of not knowing what to expect. In the interview when Isabel was a child she said:

> *I would like to know more about deaf children and possibly meet more deaf children – more deaf people as far as that goes.*

She felt that people did not understand about deafness, and said:

> *People are not quite sure what to do about her. It's not that they mean to be, they don't mean to be that way, they don't know how to go on. The truth of the matter is that there is not enough known about deafness. The general public, they don't know enough about it.*
> *(DCF, p. 196)*

In the later interview, Isabel's mother again spoke of the lack of general understanding and awareness of deafness, this time with respect to parents of newly diagnosed deaf children:

> *I have been saying this for 21 years. There should be someone they can talk to who has probably had and brought up a deaf child. Yes. Because I know that would have helped me. But when I suggested it once it was pooh-poohed and they didn't want to know. And as I said to the surgeon, an ear nose and throat surgeon, 'in your wildest dreams you can't imagine the way I feel. That's true.'*

Isabel herself felt that most hearing people did not understand about deafness and deaf people. She said:

> *I want hearing people to learn about deaf people. Hearing culture is different from Deaf culture and hearing people don't understand that.*

This book is an attempt to provide insights into deafness, to describe what it is like to grow up as a deaf person and to consider the experience of hearing parents with deaf sons and daughters. Rather than being written from a professional perspective, it seeks, by using interview data, to reflect the views of deaf young people and their families. It is based on three sets of interviews. The families were originally interviewed in the 1970s, when their deaf sons and daughters were six years old or less. Further interviews were carried out with the same families, and with the young deaf men and women themselves, in the late 1980s, some 18 years later. The study reported here considers the whole period of growing up, and the way in which attitudes have changed over that time. It also examines the continuities and discontinuities between early behaviour, experience and later life. Such personal accounts allow a consideration of more general issues in deafness, as well as challenging commonly held assumptions in the hearing world.

The information is also particularly significant for hearing families with deaf sons and daughters. One of the enduring memories of the research interviews with the parents was that at the end of the interview they were offered the opportunity to ask any question they liked. Many asked 'Are we like other families?'

Isabel and her family were part of the group that was interviewed for this book. We have started with a description of their experiences, not because they are necessarily typical of all those interviewed, for as we shall see the lives of the young people and those of their families are diverse and varied, but because her experiences illustrate many of the issues that arise for young deaf people and their families and which are the concern of this book. She talked of her own feelings about being deaf, her developing identity as a deaf person, her hopes for the future in terms of personal life and career. Her family described the shock of finding out she was deaf, their fears that she may never be able to cope, the difficulties they experienced in bringing her up, and their feelings about her growing independence. They also talked about the decisions that had to be made concerning language and communication, discipline, education and work. Her mother spoke on a number of occasions about the lack of information generally available about deafness, something which we hope this book will remedy.

The account of Isabel and her family illustrates one of the major themes of the book: language and communication. While Isabel is linguistically competent, like many deaf people she finds it difficult to understand spoken English and her speech is not easily understood by those who do not know her. This has implications for communication within the family, for education, work and social life, all of which are considered in the book. Some of the deaf young people described in the book developed spoken language, some sign language and some both; with varying degrees of competence. Because of the difficulty in accessing spoken language and because sign language was not widely available to them, particularly when they were young, some of the young people in the book do not have Isabel's linguistic competence, and the implications of this are discussed.

After the shock of the initial diagnosis, Isabel's family gradually came to accept that she was deaf. For other families it was much more difficult to come to terms with the deafness, and some families felt their lives to be blighted. One mother, for example, when asked what she enjoyed about her son, said, 'there's never been a good day with him, not one'.

Isabel had an active social life with both deaf and hearing friends, although she generally preferred the company of deaf people. Isabel identified with other deaf people, and felt she was a member of a Deaf community which she felt differed from the hearing world. Other young deaf people whom we interviewed elected to spend most of their time in the hearing world, some feeling that their deafness made little difference to their lives. As one young woman said, 'I have never regarded myself as different'. Yet others felt that they belonged nowhere. As one deaf young man said, 'I don't fit into a hearing world and I don't fit into a deaf one'.

The young people differed also in the extent of their hearing loss. Isabel would be described as severely deaf, meaning she could hear loud noises such as a large lorry passing by, but not the sound of the human voice. Others could hear voice and use the phone, while others could hear almost nothing at all. Although the extent of the hearing loss cannot be disregarded, we ourselves are not happy with a classification of this group simply in terms of what they cannot hear, for reasons to be explained later in this chapter. It is the consequences of deafness, rather than the degree of hearing loss, that are more important.

However, there is one important element that these families have in common. The young people were all born deaf, or became deaf very early in life. This sets them apart from people who become deaf later in life, when they have already learnt the spoken language of their community. Most people's experience of deaf people will be of this latter group, for while in the UK at present there are 50 000 to 70 000 individuals who were born deaf, the total population with a hearing loss is around 7.7 million, and for 2.3 million of these, the loss is likely to have a significant effect on their day-to-day lives (Institute of Hearing Research quoted by the Department of Health and Social Security (DHSS), 1988).

This chapter introduces the book, identifies some of the issues that will be discussed, and describes changes in society which have affected the lives of deaf people over the past 20 years. It also looks at the research methodology in some detail and discusses the use of interviews as a research tool. The second chapter focuses on the issue of communication by looking at communication within the family. In the following three chapters we move into the public domain by looking at school and education, work, and communication in the wider context. In Chapter 6, we return to more private worlds and consider the social lives and friendships of the deaf young people. Chapter 7 discusses what it is like to grow up as a deaf person, how the deaf young people feel about themselves and their developing deaf identity. Chapter 8 examines the impact of deafness on family life and explores in some detail the relationship between early experience and later life. The final chapter presents an overview of the whole book and returns to the major themes and issues raised in Chapter 1.

THE CONTEXT OF THE STUDY

One of the important characteristics of a book such as this, is that it provides an opportunity to look at the way in which childhood experiences, attitudes and behaviour relate to later life. Yet the period of time covered by this book has been one of great change in attitudes to deafness, and in the legislative structures and social policy that affect the lives of deaf people. Although in the book our focus is on personal experience and we hope for the most part to allow the contributions from the parents and young people to speak for themselves, it seems necessary in this first chapter to consider aspects of the wider context in which deaf young people grow up and the changes over the period of time covered by this study.

Language, communication and deafness

A major issue for hearing parents, with daughters and sons who are born deaf or become deaf early in life, is the development of language and communication. Although for some of this group hearing aids do much to make spoken language accessible, for others access to spoken language is difficult. At the time when these families were first interviewed, the dominant ideology was oralism. Parents were encouraged to use speech with their children and to try to develop their speech through the use of hearing aids and attention to lip-reading skills.

Since that time there have been conflicting influences on our approach to deaf children. The oral approach appeared to fail a significant number of children. In a classic study reported in 1979, Conrad demonstrated that for half of all those leaving educational provision for deaf children at 16 years of age, their speech was effectively unintelligible or very difficult to understand, their lip-reading skills were no better than those of hearing pupils who had not had specific training in the skill, and the median reading age was nine years (Conrad, 1979). At the same time, sign languages, which until then had been seen by many as crude systems of mime and gesture, came to be recognised as having the full linguistic properties and potential of other spoken languages. Different countries have their own unique sign languages and the sign language of the UK is British Sign Language (BSL), a term that was first used in 1975 (see Brennan, 1976). In 1988, the European Parliament recognised all European sign languages. This developing understanding of the status of sign language, together with research findings indicating that deaf children of deaf parents were more successful in language development and some academic measures, led to increasing attention being given to the potential role of sign languages in the early development of language with deaf children.

However, during this time, developments in hearing-aid technologies meant that the goal of spoken language development for deaf children through speech and hearing seemed all the more possible. Moreover, the development of cochlear implants, a sophisticated form of hearing aid which is actually implanted into the inner ear providing a perception of sound, has focused attention on the remediation of deafness. Although cochlear implants are currently limited, both in the population for which they are appropriate and in their ability to restore normal hearing, their development and the ensuing publicity with its claims of a 'bionic cure for deafness' have had an impact on debates about the appropriate language for deaf children and young people.

Education

Attitudes to sign languages have had an impact on educational policy with deaf children, as have more general changes in the educational arena in terms of general changes in educational policy and practice. The types of educational provision available for deaf children throughout this period were:

(a) Special schools, where all pupils are deaf and the approach may be oral or incorporate sign language.

(b) Partially Hearing Units (PHUs) or resourced schools, which involve groups of deaf children being educated in ordinary (mainstream) schools. In a PHU they are educated in a class group, although most spend time in classes with hearing children. In the resourced school, the deaf pupils are seen as part of the main school, but with support from specialised staff and with special provision for withdrawing them for some of the time. The approach may be entirely oral or include sign language.

(c) Integration, in which deaf pupils attend their local mainstream school or another suitable school and are educated alongside hearing pupils, usually with visits from teachers of the deaf. We have used the term 'integration' here and throughout the book, as it is the term used in the UK and by young people and parents. However, it cannot be assumed that because a deaf pupil is receiving integrated education they are fully involved with the hearing pupils, as the term itself may seem to imply. The approach is almost always oral, although a minority of integrated deaf children are educated in sign language through the provision of an interpreter.

(d) A few deaf children are educated in other special schools or units, for example those designed for children with physical disabilities or learning difficulties.

During the period covered by this book there has been a shift from placing deaf children in special schools to placing them in mainstream schools, firstly through PHUs and more recently through integration. The initial shift was from special schools to PHUs, and while in 1970, in England and Wales, there were 212 PHUs, by 1980 there were 500 (National Deaf Children's Society, 1971, 1982). The number of pupils in special schools declined in this period from 5781 in 1972 to 4847 in 1980 with a further steep decline to 3808 in 1983 (quoted in Lynas, 1986). The 1980s saw a shift to integrated education not only for deaf pupils but also for all those with special needs, formalised in the 1981 Education Act, which was implemented in 1983. It established the principle that 'all children for whom the Local Education Authority (LEA) decides to determine that special educational provision be made () are to be educated in ordinary schools in so far as is reasonably practicable' (Department of Education and Science (DES)), 1981. While in the early 1970s it was unusual for a deaf child to be integrated, a survey for the NDCS in 1987 showed that nearly three-quarters of deaf children of school age, supported by Teachers of the Deaf, in England Scotland and Wales, were educated in mainstream schools.

Not only the location of the education of deaf children changed over the period, but also the educational approach. There has been a shift from the strong oral policy of the period until the 1970s, to the greater use of sign language in schools. The first move was to Total Communication, described by Denton (1976) as comprising 'the full spectrum of language modes, child directed gesture, the language of signs, speech reading, finger spelling, reading and writing () the development of residual hearing for the enhancement of speech and speech reading skills'. In practice this has often been realised as an approach where speech and signs are used together, sometimes known as Sign Supported English (SSE). Here English is spoken and signs taken from the vocabulary of BSL are used at the same time. The results of this approach in education have been equivocal and more recently approaches using full BSL have been developed, taking a bilingual approach to the education of deaf children in which both English and BSL are seen as having a unique and separate contribution to make.

All these changes were occurring as the young people in this study passed through the education system, and these affected both the events that happened to them and the way they were described by both parents and young people.

The Deaf community

Within society as a whole, deafness is usually seen as a major handicap or disability. Deafness is viewed primarily as the inability to hear, to participate in conversations, to appreciate music or birds singing or to be aware of sound warnings of danger. This is not surprising, because most people with a hearing loss come from the group of people who become deaf with age and gradually have more and more difficulty hearing. The book describes a different group, who are born deaf or become deaf early in life, and the issues are different. They are not a group who have lost the ability to hear the spoken word or music or the birds singing – these things may have never been part of their lives or have functioned in a different way from that in the lives of hearing people.

While for some adults who were born deaf, understanding of their deafness is also based on notions of loss or impairment, for others, however, being deaf is an integral part of their being. They do not see deafness as impaired hearing, but see themselves as having a Deaf identity, as part of a community that has its own language, in this case, BSL. The recognition of BSL has given Deaf people not only a pride in their own language, but also a sense of their own identity as Deaf people, as part of a community with its own history, culture and customs (Gregory 1993). As in other minority groups, the Deaf community has recently been recon-structing its history from within (Jackson, 1991). Some members of the Deaf community now reject the idea that they are disabled and assert that they are members of a linguistic minority group. To emphasise this cultural identification, they refer to themselves as 'Deaf' rather than 'deaf'. The implications of these different notions of deafness for deaf young people and their families will be discussed in the book.

INTERVIEWING DEAF YOUNG PEOPLE AND THEIR FAMILIES

Interviewing is not an unproblematic way of obtaining information about people's lives and experiences. Even when a language and culture is shared, people's views and opinions do not exist pre-formed and ready to emerge in answer to the interviewer's questions. Interviewing deaf young people, even in their preferred language and modality, can reveal misguided assumptions on the part of the interviewer and misperceptions on the part of the young person. The remainder of this chapter and the related appendices (Appendices I, II, III) set out in some detail the issues involved in re-contacting a group of families after 18 years and in carrying out interviews with them. We felt it necessary to do this in some detail for, while superficially a consideration of research methodology may seem simply to concern procedural matters, in essence the section addresses issues that are critical to the study and to an understanding of the results.

In this section, we look in some detail at the families involved in the study, how they came to be selected, how contact was re-established after some 18 years and who was lost through this process. We also look at the construction of the final sample, and the procedures for carrying out the interviews. We consider which interviews were able to be included in the formal, quantitative analysis and those that were excluded from this, with the consequence that some of the young people are not fully represented in the results. Unlike other similar studies we have decided not to describe the young people in terms of their hearing loss and we examine the factors that contributed to this. The young people are described by their preferred form of communication and we discuss what is meant by this. We also present some basic information concerning the communication competence of the young people. A summary of this information and demographic details of the sample are presented in Appendix II.

Contacting the sample

The research study is based on interviews with 82 parents of young deaf people and 71 young deaf people themselves. Not all the interviews are included in all the quantitative analyses for reasons which are outlined below. However, the discussion and quotes utilise all of them.

The parents

In the early 1970s one of the authors, Susan Gregory, interviewed 122 mothers, and sometimes fathers, of preschool deaf children. The sample was drawn from all children, in five local authority areas, diagnosed as deaf at the time of the study.

In designing the present study it was decided to attempt to contact 101 of the original sample, the initial contact being made with the parents. The reasons for excluding 21 of the original sample are discussed in detail below. Of the 101 families, 91 (90%) were traced. Contacts were made in a number of ways, by tracing through the original address, through schools, deaf clubs, personal contacts. Once we had made a few contacts, they often led us on to others. For some of the more elusive families we scanned telephone directories and electoral rolls. Occasionally the directory enquiry service was persuaded to help. The high success rate is probably due to the perseverance of Juliet Bishop, who became skilled in exploiting the slightest lead.

Of the 91 families located, the parent or parents from 83 (82%) of the families were interviewed. Three of the families were not included as deafness was not their main concern, because the young person had severe over-riding disabilities and their parents at the initial contact suggested that much of the interview would be irrelevant to their situation. In a further two families we contacted at this stage, we were told that the child had been found not to be deaf, at a time after the first interview. In the other three families that were contacted but not interviewed, one family had emigrated and in another at the time of contact the father was seriously ill. In the third case, the young person had died in a road accident; the family were asked whether or not they wanted to be interviewed but declined.

Of the 83 interviews, only 82 could be used in the analysis, as in one interview it emerged that the young person had, in addition to his deafness, profound learning difficulties and was cared for in a residential institution. Most of the interview was not relevant to his situation. He is thus more appropriately considered with those with over-riding disabilities and to all intents and purposes he can be added to that group of exclusions, giving four in all.

We do not have any reason to feel that the ten families that were not traced introduced any obvious major systematic bias to the sample. An examination of data from the original study shows this group consisted of the families of five girls and five boys. Functional hearing loss as assessed at that time was across the range, with a slight bias to the less deaf (severely deaf 3, moderately deaf 5, partially hearing 1, loss unassessed 1). The social class distribution, as classified then, reflected that of the original sample.

The young people

Of the 82 families contacted where parents were interviewed, 71 of the young people were interviewed. Four young people were not interviewed because the parents made it clear to us in their interview that the young person's communication skills were limited in such a way as to preclude the possibility of interviewing. Six were not interviewed because the young person refused or all attempts to arrange an interview failed. In one situation the parents refused on behalf of the young person. While most of the refusals (6/7) seemed to arise from the young people themselves, our feeling is that some parents may have influenced their son's or daughter's decision not to take part; that while happy to talk themselves, they were not so happy for their son or daughter to participate. In only one instance did the parent expressly refuse on behalf of the young person, and in this situation the mother would only take part herself if we promised to make no attempt to contact her son. She felt that he was emotionally unstable and that to discuss his deafness with him would induce total depression in him. We felt we had no option but to comply.

The exclusions from the study

Three particular groups were excluded from the main study.

(a) The initial pilot sample drawn from another area (six families), who would have been more difficult to contact, as we ourselves had only limited contacts in that area, making follow up much more problematic. In fact one of those families did contact us on their own initiative, because they had heard about the study, and we interviewed the mother and her son. Parts of these interviews are quoted, but they are not included in the statistical analysis.

(b) A child who was fostered at the time of the original interview. Firstly, it would probably have been difficult to trace him, and secondly, it was likely that his parenting would not have been continuous over the period.

(c) A significant exclusion from the main analysis, and one that give us particular concern, was those families from minority ethnic groups (14 families in the original sample). This was not because we did not feel they were of concern; they are probably more worthy of attention because they are so often invisible. Initially we planned not to interview them at all for three main reasons. In the original research the interviews conducted with these families were inadequate, because of failure to take proper account of language and cultural issues. The data obtained were excluded from much of the original analysis and thus not available for comparison. Secondly, we were not convinced that our interview could adequately or appropriately touch on issues of concern to these families. Thirdly, while we felt the indigenous population would be adequately represented in such a follow-up study, changes in the constitution of the minority ethnic population meant that, even if we were able to interview these families, the fact that they would only be drawn from those present in the UK in the early 1970s would introduce bias with respect to this group.

As the research proceeded we became increasingly concerned that this group was not represented, particularly as they form a significant part of the population of young deaf people and raise crucial issues relating to attitude and policy. Also, a study of Asian families with young deaf children based on the original research, by Meherali, had yielded important results indicating the significance of deafness in a different cultural context (Meherali, 1984). We thus decided to contact those families that we could and interview them using the basic schedule but with some flexibility.

We were able to contact six families from the original sample of 14; in four instances we spoke to both parents and young person, in two to only the mother. Two families were originally from Jamaica and four were Asian families and part of the Asian community in a Midlands city with a large Asian population. We have included extracts from these interviews, but they do not form part of the statistical analysis for the reasons given above. We appreciate that this is in some sense a token approach and that the families we managed to contact are not representative of the minority ethnic population as a whole, but we hope this way at least to identify some of the important issues. We hope this will lead to a more appropriate study in the future, which is properly able to consider young deaf people and their families in the context of language and culture of ethnic minority groups.

It should also be noted that there are no deaf young people with deaf parents in the study. This is because none were brought to our attention at the time of the previous study, perhaps reflecting their different relationship with the education service at that time. (A parallel study to the initial study was, however, carried out by Gillian Hartley of deaf parents and their deaf children, employing different ways of contacting the families (Hartley, 1988)).

The interview

The parents

The interviews with the parents were carried out using a guided interview schedule, as were the previous interviews. (The use of the interview as a research tool is discussed in more detail in Appendix III.)

The 82 parent interviews were carried out with the parents of 48 young men and 34 young women. The age of the young people at the time of the parent interview was between 18 and 24 years, although 71% fell into the age range 20–22 years. It was the families themselves who decided who would take part in the interview: in 39 interviews we talked to one parent (this included step-parents, foster parents, and in one instance a sister) and in the other 43, two. Overall, our concern was to talk to someone who had intimate knowledge of the young person throughout their lives. The interviews took between one and six hours, and six required two visits. However, the vast majority, three-quarters of the interviews (63, 77%), took between two and fours hours and needed only one session.

The interviews were audio-recorded, transcribed and eventually coded. The coding schedule was devised after the majority of the interviews had been carried out, as to do this at an earlier stage could have distorted the interview process by limiting response expectations. Where appropriate, responses were then classified into particular categories, for ease of statistical manipulation.

The young people

The interviews were with 31 young women and 40 young men. The interviews with the young people were always carried out after those with the parents and usually within six months. All except one were completed in one session. Two languages were involved, as some used BSL (British Sign Language) and others English, either oral or SSE (Sign Supported English). Some used a combination of languages and modes. The deaf young people had varying degrees of facility with language and some had not been provided with the opportunity to develop their skills fully. Thus the conduct and language of the interview was an issue.

With the young people, it was clear that the interview procedure could not be the same as with the parents. Firstly, the language and mode of communication used at the interview would need to take account of the communication preference of the young person, and would vary. Secondly, we were aware that the young people themselves would have different degrees of communication competence. Thirdly, the recording procedure could not be the same, as audio-recording could not be used.

Because of the first two of these factors, the decision as to who should carry out the interviews was not straightforward. We considered, but rejected, the idea of having a number of different interviewers to meet the different requirements of individual interviews. However, we decided on only one interviewer as we felt it important to maintain some consistency, and we wanted an interviewer who could be fully involved throughout the research. We felt that the person who did the interviews should be deaf themselves, and we could have elected to choose a deaf person whose first language was BSL. However, pure BSL would be inappropriate for many of the sample, as we knew that they all started out with an oral approach, and had been introduced to English at school. While some would have acquired BSL later on, only one came from a family where some BSL was used at home; for the rest, the language of the home was not BSL. We therefore felt that the choice of a deaf interviewer, whose first language was English but who also had BSL skills, was the most appropriate. All the interviews were thus carried out by one of the authors and the consultant to the project, Lesley Sheldon, who is herself deaf. Her first language is English, and her preferred means of communication is English, with signs used in support, (SSE) though she is able to communicate in BSL.

We were able to introduce some flexibility into the interview situation itself, as we decided to record the interviews using a notetaker, a second person who was present at all the interviews. We considered, but rejected, the use of a video camera, following discussions with people experienced in this technique. There is some debate about how necessary or valuable video recording is in studies involving deaf people. Our own view is that, while many adult deaf people may feel comfortable being video-recorded, it could have been intimidating for our sample of deaf young people, some of whom may have been less confident of their communication abilities. The notetakers' main task was to take as full notes as possible on the interview. They also noted whether or not questions had been repeated or re-worded and those questions that did not seem to have been understood. At the end of the interview, the notetaker and interviewer wrote additional notes on the interview based on their immediate recollection and to provide as full a record as possible.

However, the notetaker had a second function that evolved as important as the interviews progressed, which was to provide communication support. For oral deaf people the notetaker was usually a hearing person who could clarify points if necessary, and provide an extra source of information. If the person was known to prefer to use BSL, a deaf person with competence in BSL would be notetaker. Occasionally in these circumstances they would assist in actually carrying out the interview, in collaboration with the interviewer. This seemed to us to minimise the disadvantages of having only one interviewer.

We had a range of notetakers available to us, drawn from personal contacts. Some were hearing with experience of deaf people, some were hearing and qualified interpreters, or with good knowledge of sign language. Some were deaf with good literacy skills in English. The notetaker was always chosen to match the communication requirements of the deaf person as far as we could ascertain them. A series of specially devised questions was included in the interview with the parents in order to establish this.

Issues involved in interviewing deaf people as part of a research study are discussed in more detail in Appendix III.

The presentation of results

The quantitative analysis

Eighty-two parent interviews were carried out. However, at some points in the analysis, only 81 interviews could be used, as one of the interviewees was a foster mother who had limited knowledge of the child's early life. Qualitative data in the form of quotes is, however, drawn from all the interviews.

Of the 71 young people's interviews, only 61 were included in the statistical analyses. Ten had to be excluded as insufficient responses of those young people could be coded. These ten were excluded from the analysis after interview, although quotes from their interviews are used where appropriate. For the ten that were excluded, in one the interview was not attempted, and only brief conversations were carried out, mostly focused around drawings. For a further three, the interview was abandoned part way through, and for six, the interview was carried out but not coded (two) or coded and then excluded (four) as many of the answers were uncodable. The criteria for exclusion were that for 20% of the cases when responses were coded, the young person had either not understood the question or not been able to formulate an answer to it that we could make sense of, and it was not possible to code it.

A major concern is, of course, that so many of the young people could not be included in the quantitative analysis because of poor language skills. From the original 82 families involved, only 61 (74%) of the young people's responses are represented in the statistical analysis. While in seven cases this was due to non-contact or refusal of the young person to take part, the major reason was difficulties in communication. In four of the families, the responses of the parents clearly indicated the young person would not be able to take part and a further ten were excluded after they had been interviewed. Thus information from 14 of the young people in the original 82 families contacted (17%) was not included in the statistical analysis because the language of the young people was restricted in such a way as to prevent them discussing their lives and experience in detail. This represents one in six of the sample. It is worth noting here that these exclusions were young people who were described by their parents as deaf; for them the deafness was the main issue. Those instances (four) where the parents saw their son or daughter as having profound learning difficulties were excluded from the research at an earlier stage. We will return again to this group in Chapter 7, where we will give these young people special consideration.

Because we had data on fewer young people and because those with the poorest language skills had to be excluded from the quantitative analysis of the young people, where information was available from both parents and young people on a particular topic, we usually elected to present the parental data. This was, of course, providing we had no reason to believe that the parental responses differed significantly from those of the young people, either through different access to the information or through differing perspectives on the topic.

The qualitative analysis

Wherever possible we have tried to illustrate our comments with quotes from the interviews. These are taken from all the interviews, including those from families from minority ethnic groups, and not just those included in the quantitative analysis. With the parents it was possible to use verbatim quotes from the transcript of the interviews. This was not possible for the young people and in giving quotes from these we have used the notes made at the interviews. We have chosen to present them in good English that reflects as faithfully as possible the original response, whether that was initially signed or spoken. Occasionally, however, where the BSL gloss of the interview, or the verbatim quote (even if ungrammatical in a conventional sense) had more impact or was more direct, we have used this.

For example, in answer to the question, 'Do you ever feel sorry for yourself?', Ann gave a reply in BSL for which the direct gloss was *Yes because people talk to me nothing*. This seems a much more vivid response than the English translation, which would be something like 'Yes, because people don't talk to me' or 'Yes, because no-one talks to me'.

GROUP DISCUSSIONS

As well as material from the interviews, some supplementary information is included from group discussions with two groups of young people interviewed for the research. We convened these discussions for a number of reasons. Firstly, there were some issues in the interviews we wanted to probe further and secondly, we were interested to know what the young people had thought about the interview process and this would be more easily ascertained in group discussions. In addition, we did feel that some of the young people may be interested to meet other participants and share views.

Two groups each of five young people were convened. Originally the intention was to have one group conducted orally and the other through BSL, but the groups ultimately were mixed and overall there was a range of language in each group. One interpreter facilitated the first group and two the second. Notetakers were present at the groups and in addition information was obtained from audio-recordings made at the time, of the young people or the interpreter. Each group took place on a Saturday and consisted of three sessions spread throughout the day with a break for lunch.

We were pleased with the extra information we obtained and felt that for some topics the group discussion added to our understanding of the issues. Quotes from these discussions are described as such throughout the text.

THE YOUNG PEOPLE

Communication competence

As it was clear that the communication of the young people would be a critical issue for this research we endeavoured to get some measure of their skills and their ability to answer the questions on the scale. As a measure of how well the interview schedule as a whole was understood, we checked on the proportion of the interview questions that had to be rephrased at each interview for those young people included in the quantitative analysis. The results of this are shown in Table 1.1.

While it is encouraging to see that for a third of the interviewees, no questions or only a few questions had to be rephrased, it is disturbing that, for one-quarter, over half the schedule had to be rephrased. Even then, questions were not always understood or responded to appropriately. For some, there were young people who were unable to answer, or we were unable to obtain a response of which we could make sense. Therefore, many of the tables showing young people's responses do not total 61, indicating that not all the group could answer that particular question or the answer given did not make sense in terms of the question asked. This is discussed in more detail in the final chapter.

Because the ability to understand and to answer questions is important, we felt it important to have a measure of their level of understanding and comprehension. We devised a scale by selecting four questions from the schedule to indicate their understanding of straightforward questions, and four to indicate their understanding of complex questions. The questions used for these scales were:

Table 1.1. *The extent to which interview questions to young deaf people had to be rephrased*

Proportion rephrased	Number of interviews	Percentage
None	3	5
Few	19	31
Less than half	16	26
Half	8	13
More than half	15	25

General comprehension

Before you left school did you do any voluntary work, paid work or get any work experience?

Which schools did you go to?

What is your ideal partner, deaf or hearing?

If you have any problems with your relationship or with sex, who would you go to to talk about it?

Complex questions

At school, did you have any group discussions about work and relationships at work?

Were your mother and father able to explain to you about things that were going to happen?

Violence on television makes violence in real life worse? (in series of questions about attitudes)

How would life be different if you were not deaf?

In all these, the answer to each question was assessed on a three-point scale of 0–2. Zero indicated that the question was not understood, 1 indicated some understanding of the question, and 2 an understanding of the full question the first time it was asked, with no rewording. The results are shown in Table 1.2, which indicates that 59% understood virtually all general questions and 18% all the complex questions.

We also looked at their ability to give complex answers. Here the scoring system used zero for no response or an ambiguous answer where the question appeared not to have been understood. A score of 1 was used if the answer was appropriate and indicated the question had been understood but, even after prompting, the answer put forward a simple view of the topic. A score of 2 was used if the answer went beyond a basic answer and showed some complexity of thinking on the issue. The following gives the four questions used for this scale and examples of answers with their codes.

Q. Can you tell me what kind of person you are?

> *I am mostly happy.*
> *Rosemary (oral)*

Score 1

Q. Do you have any views on how deaf children should be educated?

> *Yes, in special schools for the deaf.*
> *Robert (BSL)*

Score 1

Q. All policemen should have guns?

> *No, if they did, like in America, when something happened they would be more likely to get shot. It's better without. Maybe if they know there is a dangerous man, or hostages are being held – then its OK.*
> *Paula (BSL user)*

Score 2

Q. Has there ever been a time when you wished you were hearing?

> *Yes, of course. It's really when I want information, like when I am watching television and there's no subtitles. Sometimes I do so I can join in group discussions. When I left M... (school) I wished I was hearing because I thought I would be able to cope better at University. It doesn't bother me now.*
> *Ray (oral)*

Score 2

The scores obtained are given in Table 1.2. As can be seen, about a third gave complex answers to most of the questions on the scale, and a further third gave complex answers some of the time.

Table 1.2. *Comprehension of eight interview questions and ability to give complex answers*

	0–2	3–4	5–6	7–8
General comprehension	1 (2%)	4 (7%)	20 (33%)	36 (59%)
Complex comprehension	7 (11%)	21 (34%)	22 (36%)	11 (18%)
Complex answers	3 (5%)	16 (26%)	23 (38%)	19 (31%)

Hearing loss

In much of the literature on deafness, particularly that with an educational focus, the individuals described are classified in terms of their hearing loss. After much consideration, we rejected this. Firstly, while hearing loss is a major concern of educationalists, to most other groups, and in particular to deaf people themselves, it is seen as irrelevant. Some would put it more strongly, that rather than focusing on what deaf people are and can do, it defines people in terms of their difference from the hearing community, with thus an emphasis on a deficiency model of deafness.

Secondly, the definition of hearing loss is actually complex and not as simple as the scientific trappings surrounding its measurement would suggest. Educationalists themselves distinguish between the pure tone audiometry test, which is seen as giving some absolute measure of loss, and more functional criteria in terms of the individual's ability to make sense of the sounds that they hear. It is suggested that pure audiological data tell us little of how a child actually functions. A functional criterion was used in the book detailing the results of the first interview study. This resulted in a letter of protest from at least one mother that in labelling her child as moderately hearing because he responded to voice, we did not properly reflect the work she had done with him to develop his spoken language skills. On pure tone audiology he would register a more severe loss than this description might suggest.

The third reason is the lack of available information. We did initially ask both parents and young people about the degree of hearing loss. (This was despite reservations from Lesley Sheldon, the deaf consultant to the project, and other deaf people whom we talked to in the early stages of the project.) We also attempted a functional assessment ourselves based on answers to a range of questions concerning hearing particular sounds, use of the telephone, etc. Interestingly, although the questions on the telephone were not important for classifying hearing loss, they did throw interesting light on aspects of family communication and codes surrounding the use of the telephone – see Chapter 5. Asking about degree of hearing loss confirmed the irrelevance of such categories for most deaf people and their families.

Often in answers to questions about hearing loss, the information they were given about decibel loss was expressed inappropriately as a percentage loss.

> *He has 20% hearing in one ear.*
> *Mother of Clive, 20 years, BSL*

Often the young people too gave figures for a percentage loss.

> *Seventy-nine to eighty-five per cent.*
> *Mark, 20 years, oral*

> *No hearing in the left ear and 70% in the right.*
> *Geoffrey, 21 years, oral*

Others were confused.

> *I am profoundly partially deaf.*
> *Shaun, 21 years, BSL*

> *I am profoundly deaf but some say I am partially deaf.*
> *Bobby, 20 years, SSE*

> *He is dumbfoundly deaf.*
> *Mother of Guy, 21 years, LLS (LLS defined below)*

Others were clearly not concerned about such categorisation.

> *All I know is I'm deaf.*
> *Louise, 22 years, oral*

> *I don't know, I think I have a chart at home.*
> *Ruth, 19 years, oral*

> *I've no idea and I am not interested.*
> *Trevor, 22 years, oral*

The responses of the parents and the young people to the questions concerning hearing loss are shown in Table 1.3. Apart from some agreement on the use of the term 'profoundly deaf' (which in fact over-represented that group with respect to other studies), the agreement was small between the two groups. In asking the question, we ourselves of course gave credibility to the notion that it was relevant, which may have put pressure on the young people to come up with an answer.

Table 1.3. *Degrees of hearing loss reported by parents and young people*

	Parents		Young people	
	Number	%	Number	%
Profound	52	63	32	53
Severe	9	11	4	7
Moderate	0	0	1	2
Partially hearing	9	11	7	12
Don't know	12	15	15	25
Not answered	0	0	2	3

This lack of knowledge about hearing loss has been reported in other studies. Phoenix (1988) in a study of deaf adults in Northern Ireland used a functional definition of loss, because 'the research team knew that deaf people rarely understand how deaf they are in terms of "decibel loss"'. This was also apparent in another study (Silo, work in progress) of deaf teachers, who, as a group working in education, are familiar with the categories. The replies received included:

I don't know, I don't bother, I just know I'm deaf.

People ask me what my hearing loss is. I feel it is personal and not relevant. After all, I do not ask friends who wear glasses what their sight loss is...this is a dilemma that is unresolved. What do other deaf teachers do?

We therefore decided that in most of the book we would not describe the young people in this way. Overall we felt that for the young people such a distinction was of little relevance and to use it would impose an artificial distinction emphasising deficiency. However, we do accept that in terms of educational attainments hearing loss has a specific predictive value. We were also interested to see whether it influenced school placement, and decisions about educational approach. Therefore, occasionally, in particular contexts we make reference to hearing loss. For this we use the functional assessment derived from the parent interview as giving the most complete and up-to-date information. For the most part, however, we reflect the attitude of our interviewees and pay no regard to it.

The preferred language of the young people

Whilst we rejected hearing loss as an appropriate descriptive category, we did feel it would be useful to provide information about the young people

Table 1.4. *Preferred language of the*
young people

	Number	%
BSL	31	38
SSE	13	16
Oral	30	37
LLS	8	10

when we quoted their views. We felt the category of preferred language would be useful here as indicating a positive choice on the part of the young person and indicating the group with which they identified. These categories were based for the most part on the information given at the interviews with the young people themselves and usually reflected both the language and mode of the interview. We were generous in our attribution of language and the category does not imply fluency in the language but the use of a recognisable linguistic form. In all cases where the young person was interviewed, we based our attribution of preferred language on information obtained at the interview. This included those whose interviews could not be coded. Where the young person was not interviewed, the preferred language had to be based on information obtained in the parent interviews (11 instances).

We did find we had to introduce a category of 'limited language skills' (LLS) where it was impossible, in the face-to-face situation, to use any linguistic form, or when the information from the parents indicated a lack of useful language. This was used for eight young people overall, four where the parents suggested that an interview would not be possible, and four where we visited but could not interview. In the case of parental information, we only used the category if there was no person with whom the young person was described as having a relationship in which some language-based communication was used, and it does not simply reflect parental inability to communicate with them. For some we interviewed, we could establish a preferred language even if the interview could not be coded. The numbers in each category are shown in Table 1.4.

A significant number of those who were oral, or used SSE, were starting to learn to sign, although they were not yet fluent. Because of difficulties in defining bilinguality, and because we did not want to introduce an assessment of bilingual skills into the interview, we have no detailed figures on the number who were competent in each language or who aspired to be. Our impression is, however, that at the time of the interview 44 were bilingual in the sense that they actively used two languages in their

Table 1.5. *Preferred language and hearing loss*

	BSL	SSE	Oral	LLS
Profound	17	7	2	5
Severe	12	5	12	1
Moderate	2	1	8	2
Partial	0	0	8	0

day-to-day lives. Of those who were not bilingual, eight were BSL users, one an SSE user, 21 were oral and eight had limited language skills. Clearly none of those with limited language skills could be bilingual, and two-thirds of those who were oral (21/31, 68%) had not developed BSL skills. Nearly all the SSE users were bilingual (12/13, 92%) and the young woman who was not, was among those whose interview could not be coded. The eight BSL users who did not use English, either spoken or written in their day-to-day lives, had poor literacy skills and two were among those whose interviews could not be used in the quantitative analysis. As might be expected there was some relationship between preferred language and hearing loss, as is shown in Table 1.5. All those who were partially hearing were oral, and those who were profoundly deaf varied in their preferred language but were more likely to prefer BSL than were those who were moderately deaf, who were more likely to be oral. Equal numbers of those who were severely deaf were oral or used BSL.

Gender differences

Table 1.6 shows the relationship between gender and preferred language. All those with limited language skills were male, but even when they are excluded, there was a significant relationship between preferred language and gender ($\chi^2 = 10.90$, $p < 0.01$) with young men more likely to be oral and young women more likely to use SSE. This is not a language difference, as SSE is English-based, thus there were 23 young men and 20 young women who communicated using a form of English. It seems that young women who use English are more likely to accompany it with signs taken from BSL. The proportions adopting BSL were similar (17/48, 35% men, 14/34, 41% women). There was, however, no clear relationship between hearing loss and gender; see Table 1.7.

Table 1.6. *Preferred language and gender*

	BSL	SSE	Oral	LLS
Young men	17	2	21	8
Young women	14	11	9	0

Table 1.7. *Gender and hearing loss*

	Profoundly deaf	Severely deaf	Moderately deaf	Partially hearing
Young men	15	17	11	5
Young women	16	13	2	8

CONCLUSION

In this chapter we have described in some considerable detail the sample interviewed, and the language skills of the young people interviewed. We were delighted with the number of families we were able to contact after such a long period of time and extremely grateful to the families for the time they gave to speak to us and the frankness of their answers.

However, we do feel concern at the linguistic competence of some of the young people. Although many of them were articulate and competent communicators and gave us much food for thought, there was a minority who did not have adequate skills to participate fully in the interview. Some of these had limited language skills in any language. We will return to this issue at various points throughout the book.

In many ways this may appear to be a depressing book. It paints a picture of families under stress, of young people who are not fully participating in society and of unrealised potential. However, if this gives the reader a negative view of deafness or of the families this would be a serious error. We have enjoyed meeting these young deaf people and their families. They have been generous with their time and shared with us in many intimate details of their lives, some of which have been stressful for them to discuss. We are immensely grateful for this. With many of the young people we have been impressed by their attitudes, by their enthusiasm for life, by their resilience and by their lack of resentment of the misunderstanding and marginalisation that they have encountered. With the parents we have been challenged by their insights and impressed by the sensitive and reflective way they have discussed their sons' and daughters' lives. Many have themselves said how having a deaf child has made them think deeply, in ways that they may not otherwise have done, about bringing up children and the attitudes of society in general. We ourselves hope that the book, rather than confirming deafness as a personal tragedy, challenges both the Deaf community and hearing world to be more constructive and positive in their approach to deaf young people and their families so that young deaf people may realise their full potential.

CHAPTER TWO

Family life and communication

It is really great when we (the family) all get together, but last week we got together for the first time in ages, months and months. I couldn't handle it because we all got excited, we all wanted to talk at once, and I couldn't follow them. I got a bit upset because I said 'you are the closest members of the family, the closest to me, but I am having to struggle to understand what is going on. I don't feel I should have to struggle in the family – maybe outside, but not in the family'.
Janet, 22 years, oral

In general, as sons and daughters move through their teens and into adult life the relationship with the parents develops and changes. Often during adolescence there are periods when the relationship is fraught and many see this as a necessary part of the evolving relationship. By the time early adulthood is reached, however, the relationships become more stable and this seemed the case for many in the sample. As with hearing families, topics of conversation varied from family to family.

We have a good relationship – we talk about everything.
Tina, 18 years, oral

We chat about my getting married and so on, but if I try to talk more deeply my mother brushes it off.
Marion, 19 years, BSL

I don't talk to them about my private life though.
Francis, 19 years, oral

The young people quoted above were describing their relationship with their parents. As would be expected the whole range of relationships was represented in the sample from very close to estranged, although it would be fair to say that the vast majority of parent–son or daughter relationships were positive with varying degrees of intimacy. But an integral aspect of such relationships must be communication and, as the quote that heads this chapter indicates, communication within the family was not always straightforward, an issue we explore in this chapter.

When their children were of preschool age, the majority of parents (76%) had described their main problem with their child to be communication and even more (89%) saw that to be the main difficulty from their child's point of view. Eighteen years later just over half the parents in the study still claimed to be concerned about their son's or daughter's communication skills; over half of these 'extremely' so.

Aspects of the process of communication affected the dynamics of family life. In this chapter we look at these issues in more detail and ask whether this is inevitable for hearing families with deaf offspring. For the most part the families had worked hard to achieve a good relationship; they had followed advice they had been given. They had often reflected upon their situation and been conscious of communication to a far greater extent than occurs in families where all the members are hearing. For hearing parents of hearing children, shared communication is simply a means to an end. Untaught and incidentally, language develops so that the means of communication can be taken for granted. For many of the deaf young people and their families, the development of communication itself was an issue.

COMMUNICATION WITHIN THE FAMILY

I want to laugh at the same time as the others.

An area of major concern for both the deaf young people and their parents was the dynamics of communication when there were larger groups of people involved. The major issues seemed to arise when the family came together as a group.

> *When I talk to Mum its all right, but if the family or someone interrupts, my mother does not finish what we are talking about. I say to her that I was talking to you first but when I try to talk to Mum or get in on the conversation, they tell me to wait.*
> *Marion, 19 years, BSL*

Many young people, as the above quote indicates, felt hurt at the way they could be excluded in such settings.

I always felt left out at family get-togethers. They did not often try to tell me what was being said – so I had to ask them. I don't visit the family at all now, only for weddings and special things.
Nicky, 21 years, SSE

If I can't follow I get angry, I say 'I'm here'. At Christmas I get bored, I ask them what they've said. () It's the same now; nothing has changed. I keep telling them, but they can't think about me all the time.
Interviewer: Could your family improve their communication with you?
Yes. They could try and include me more and not pretend that I am part of the furniture. They should offer to tell me what they are saying.
Tina, 18 years, oral

I can't follow the talk. I feel a bit angry and frustrated. If I ask them what they are talking about they say 'wait a bit', and then they don't tell me what they are talking about.
Marion, 19 years, BSL

In many families, conscious attempts were made to fully involve the deaf person.

Even in family gatherings now I find myself interrupting people and saying to Carol 'Did you hear what Aunty Vi said?' and if she says 'No' then I go over it all again and make them wait until I have let Carol know, so they realise they must include her as well. After all these years we are still doing it.
Mother of Carol, 23 years, oral

The effort made by this family led the father to reflect what it must be like for his daughter.

Father: I think that in all fairness to Carol, you just don't appreciate her difficulties. This is the sobering thing, that we have had a deaf daughter for about 23 years and I don't think really that possibly we have the basic understanding of what she feels like.
Mother: I don't see how you can tell, because unless you have been deaf yourself you have got no clue.
Father: I think it's so sad, because we tend to look at everything from our own standpoint () the effort that she has got to make just to remain

in a conversation and pick things up that we take for granted.
Parents of Carol, 23 years, oral

But, however much the family was sensitive to the needs of the deaf person, it was not ideal, for no one likes to disrupt the whole conversation. As Phillip said, in the quote that heads this section, when describing how his family always explained any jokes to him that had been made at table.

I want to laugh at the same time as the others.
Phillip, 19 years, SSE

And sometimes, attempts by family members to involve the young deaf person were seen as patronising.

I can't remember any times (good times with the family) because a family party is not ideal for me. I never talk, I just listen. People say 'Hello', 'How are you?' or 'Sunday dinner – OK?' that's all.
Nigel, 19 years, oral

It raises the issue as to whether such communication difficulties are inevitable. An interesting comment on this is raised by the following two excerpts from an interview with Paula, who contrasted the frustration of conversation with her parents with the ease of communication with her friends.

I get frustrated. If I try and interrupt they say, 'Wait a minute'. I sometimes shout at my Mum and Dad because they do not understand how I feel.

And later in the same interview:

Lots of friends (deaf) stay here now and we chat all the time. Now my mother and father feel left out so they know how I felt.
Paula, 24 years, BSL

These quotes make an important point. This deaf young woman had lively and interesting conversations with her friends, yet when she was together with her family she often felt left out. Yet this was a family with a genuine concern for their daughter and where relationships between family members were strong and supportive. Clearly, her deafness of itself was not a barrier to lively and stimulating conversation, as evidenced by her easy communication with her deaf friends. Anyone who spends time with groups of deaf people or families where all the members are deaf can testify to the fact that communication can be lively and uninhibited. This point is discussed again later in the chapter.

You can't catch the moment

Communication in the one-to-one situation was usually easier. The stressful situation described by the young person at the head of the chapter was not typical of her one-to-one conversations within her family.

> *Mum and Dad have always listened to what I have got to say. ( ) I discuss with my Dad sometimes about me being deaf and what problems I have, how I am doing at work and he is very interested. I talk to my parents about politics, what is on the television and what they think about philosophy. I don't have complications now.*
> Janet, 22 years, oral

Yet, although for many of the young people and their parents, one-to-one conversations were fine, for some they were just not adequate, and it was not possible to talk over those things that they felt it was important to discuss.

> *He misunderstands a lot. He thinks I am talking down to him a lot. He says 'you make me feel small' and it is a complete misunderstanding. I am not doing that at all and I don't understand what he means when he says that to me. Talking things out, he finds he has not got the patience to sit and talk problems out. He gets upset unnecessarily; if he would stop and talk.*
> Mother of Colin, 24 years, BSL

> *I think the worst time is when he is upset, and he has to explain himself, what he feels inside. When Pamela died, he did cry, but he couldn't explain his feelings. It was difficult to get through to him.*
> Mother of Bobby, 20 years, SSE

There were other difficulties. For many parents, sadness lay in their own appreciation of what the deaf young person was missing in terms of incidental conversation, asides, overhead conversations and 'chats'.

> *You can't carry on a normal conversation. It's giving that instant comment, you can't catch the moment. By the time you have got his attention the situation might have passed. He doesn't say he misses anything, but he wouldn't know if he missed anything.*
> Mother of Ray, 21 years, oral

The issue could arise over not understanding the nuances in conversation as even when communication was well established some of the subtleties could be lost.

He can't understand the tone in a voice. He never has been able to understand sarcasm. He doesn't hear that change in the tone of voice, and he doesn't know what it means. He only hears the sentence; it's like talking on a level all the time. Your voice does not go up or down; it's unfair to speak to him in any other way than straight meaning.
Father of Alistair, 21 years, oral

She doesn't know the meaning of a joke; if you say something, it's serious. She can't see double meaning. She'll laugh at Laurel and Hardy, it's visual; but as far as language goes, she doesn't understand, you can't play around with it.
Mother of Marion, 19 years, BSL

Further misunderstandings often arose when a mother would describe the content of a conversation the young person had observed but not participated in.

He will often say, 'What did you say?' and perhaps I have been talking for about three minutes and I tell him in a split second, and he says, 'Why have you been. . .?' and when I am on the phone to Hazel's Mum I can be on about twenty minutes and it is the same. I say well, we have been talking about the weather and he says, 'Well what did she say about the weather?'
Mother of Andrew, 21 years, BSL

They said they thought I knew already

A more insidious consequence of the difficulties in group discussion and the limits on informal conversation, however, seemed to be that many deaf young people often found that they had not been made aware of significant family events, often not until well after the event. As far as it is possible to ascertain, this rarely seemed to be due to deliberate concealment, but just that they had missed out on the information. Assumptions hearing people make as to how information is transmitted may break down where there are deaf family members.

When my cousin was expecting a baby I was the last to know about it. It was not until she was a month due. It was all at the last minute before I knew.
Interviewer: What do you feel about that?
I feel mad sometimes. I feel, 'Why didn't you tell me?' – you know. I felt annoyed sometimes.
Interviewer: Did you ask your family why they didn't tell you?

Well, my Mum, she's the one that knows everything, you know. So, she's the one that tells everybody what is happening and this and that. I asked her why and she said, 'I thought I'd told you'.
Interviewer: Did you accept that explanation?
No.
Interviewer: Why do you think she hadn't told you?
I don't know really. I just think she should have told me.
Trevor, 22 years, oral

When my father left, my mother never told me where he had gone and why.
Ann, 21 years, BSL

I had a cousin in hospital. They didn't tell me. My grandmother told me and I was angry. They said they thought I knew already.
Tina, 18 years, oral

When my grandfather died my mother never told me and I found out a lot later.
Mother of Andrew, 21 years, BSL

When the young people were asked whether there were important family matters that had not been communicated to them, of the 49 who answered the question, 39 (80% of those responding, and 64% of the total sample) said this had happened to them, although 15 of these did say that although it had happened they were not concerned about it. It is of course likely that this occurred to the majority of those who could not answer the question also.

You can't talk to him, you've got to show him.

For some families of course all the issues discussed above were magnified, as the language skills of the deaf young person were extremely limited. Some of the young people (8/82, 10%) could not be understood at all, or only in a very limited way and by a few people or just one person, often the mother. The mother of the young person quoted above described later in the interview what was meant by 'show':

I mean when he's talking about me he does (meaning gestures or mimes) my glasses. When he's talking about his sister, he does her long hair. When his brother, he'll draw a moustache.
Mother of Brian, 22 years, LLS

Another mother, whose son's interview had to be abandoned because of his limited language skills, said of the family's understanding of her son:

> *They never could. They tried but they couldn't. They didn't know what he was saying. () When he's talking to my sisters, he tells them things and they don't understand, and they've thought he's meant something else but he hasn't.*
> Mother of Matthew, 21 years, LLS

This was also an issue for one of the mothers of the young people from a minority ethnic group, who had visual difficulties as well as his deafness and had limited communication skills.

> *He can't really sign. But he loves his tummy. If he wants a biscuit or anything like that he'll do it (rub his stomach) or if he wants to go for a walk he'll (points at door). He can't communicate really, more if he wants something he'll show us.*
> Mother of Adam, 22 years, LLS

The English only speak one language, they only understand what it is like to speak one language.

Different issues were involved in three of the six families we spoke to from minority ethnic groups, where the first or main family language was not English, but Gujerati. One family had already decided before they arrived in England to speak English for the children, independently of having a deaf child, mainly because through their work they had become fluent in English, while they lived in East Africa.

> *We don't have any problem with communication, we usually speak English at home. In Africa we spoke with English people there and that's how I learnt to speak English. I could read and write English, everything.*
> *Interviewer: What other languages do you speak?*
> *I speak Gujerati, Punjabi, Swahili. I speak three or four languages. I can read Gujerati and Punjabi but I can't read Swahili. When we were in Africa they'd just started teaching Swahili.*
> Mother of Ritesh, 24 years, BSL

In another family, the family did not speak English, although the father could understand it. They were disappointed their son had not learnt to read and write to a higher level, as that would have helped communication in the family. They also wished that advice had been available to them in their own language, particularly in the early stages.

It's more difficult because they do not speak English, but they under-
stand and they try to help…It would be nice if there was more support
and more encouragement for people who can't communicate in Eng-
lish. At the beginning they would have liked more ideas and more
support on how they could help…
Mother of Kunal, 24 years, BSL (interview facilitated by Kunal's
brother's wife)

Another family had resigned themselves to having to speak English at
home, as that was the advice they were given, but with reluctance,
particularly as the mother did not feel comfortable speaking English, and
the grandfather who lived with them only spoke Gujerati.

When I speak to him, I always speak in English. She (his mother) speaks
in Gujerati but he understands. It's difficult. We feel we should speak
Gujerati at home. It is our mother tongue. So this is another problem we
face. We speak two languages at home, as one is a mother language, and
then English, which is my second language. You might say that he (Anil)
is born here, so English is his mother language, but really there is
another language, our family language, Gujerati. My father only speaks
Gujerati, but because he (Anil) is deaf we must also speak English. It
would be very difficult for him to understand two languages, you know.
Father of Anil, 23 years, BSL

While he agreed with the advice he had been given, and felt himself that
using only English with his son was beneficial, he did feel that those who
advised him so strongly on this had little understanding of the major
undertaking involved.

The English only speak one language, they only understand what it is
like to speak one language.
Father of Anil, 23 years, BSL

COMMUNICATION WITH INDIVIDUAL FAMILY MEMBERS

My father tells my mother so she can tell me

In the families described, where the communication of the young person
was extremely limited, almost invariably the only person who could
communicate with the young person at all was the mother. In other
families, too, communication was better with one family member than

others, and this was usually the mother. Sometimes the young person could only really communicate with one family member, either because they knew them the best or because they were the one that had developed the necessary skills.

> *My mother explains things to me or I explain to my mother. Sometimes my mother writes things down. I sign sometimes and sometimes I talk. My mother realises it's difficult and she can finger spell to me. If I finger spell to her she says, 'Do it again, do it again'. My father cannot sign at all, he does not understand me. My sister does not sign, she uses finger spelling and I lip read. Neil (my brother) uses finger spelling, I try to lip read him but it's too difficult, as he talks too fast. Sometimes my father tells my mother things so she can tell me.*
> *Helen, 23 years, SSE*

This young woman was able to express herself and her ideas, as can be seen from quotes from her on pages 98, 190 and 191, yet despite the efforts made within the family communication was difficult and she remained excluded except when specific attempts were made to tell her things. The responsibility for this lay with the mother.

Throughout the interviews there were many examples of difficulties in communicating with the father.

> *I talk to my mother, my father doesn't understand me. He never speaks. I don't know why.*
> *Marion, 19 years, BSL*

> *I don't bother to talk to my father – he drinks and smokes all the time. Sometimes I can't understand Mum and sometimes it's all right.*
> *Richard, 20 years, oral*

> *Well, father is a problem, he keeps his lips very stiff. He has got a stiff upper lip, and he knows that. I say to him, 'Dad, move your lips a bit more'. I think sometimes he gets a bit upset when I can't understand him. () My mother has to talk for him. 'Oh Mum, what did he say?' and I know I shouldn't do it, I don't like it. If someone is talking to me and they say, 'What did she say?' I don't like it, it's horrible. But I don't do it very often. Only when I am tired I turn to Mum, because she is easier to lip read.*
> *Janet, 22 years, oral*

> *My father is lazy, he never looks at me, because he just does not bother. Yes. Lazy () I watch him but he does not watch me. I am always teasing him because he can't see very well. My father has very little time for me*

*– he is trying to get extra time – he still worries about me because I am
deaf. He doesn't really understand.*
Josie, 24 years, BSL

*My mother is learning sign language. My father tried, but he is under a
lot of stress. My mother is teaching him.*
Zoe, 19 years, BSL

In both these last two examples the young people made excuses for their
father's poor communication. It was not unusual for the young people to
accept such limitations in this way. We were struck in a number of
situations by their tolerance of poor communication in the family.

Mothers also described the problems that fathers had with
communication.

*He doesn't understand her quite as well as the rest of us and that is
contact – the amount of time parents spend with their children, and he
doesn't spend as much time.*
Mother of Paula, 24 years, BSL

*His dad is much different. () His dad is inclined to speak very...with his
mouth...very...mumbles a bit. And he (her son) will say to me, 'What
does his mouth say?' () and I will say, 'Well ask him again' and he will
say, 'What did you say?' and he speaks it better then.*
Mother of Gavin, 19 years, oral

*Now dad, he tends, from Terry being little, to exaggerate a little bit.
You've heard of people who exaggerate and confuse. I can see Terry
looking at dad trying to work out what he's said. I can say the same
thing like I'm talking to you. He can understand what I say and he turns
to his dad, Oh! and answers. It's not all the time, but occasionally that
still happens.*
Mother of Terry, 22 years, oral

When mothers explained the reason for the poor communication of their
husbands they often described it in terms of embarrassment.

*Robert taught me, (finger spelling). And we all had a little picture of the
alphabet, all except my husband. He could never bring himself to do it.*
Interviewer: *Does he feel embarrassed?*
*I think he does. I think he does feel embarrassed. Now Robert can't
communicate with him well at all.*
Interviewer: *Does Robert feel sad about that?*
I think so, mmmm. I would if it were my father. Very sad. But he just has

not been able to bring himself to do it. He is very conscious over things like that...He is very reserved like that, always has been.
Mother of Robert, 22 years, BSL

The general impression gained from the interviews was that communication with the father was in many cases difficult. Although there was no specific question to the young people about the person in the family with whom they had the most problems communicating, almost all of those who spontaneously mentioned a family member being particularly difficult, specified the father (16/61, 26%, a quarter of the total sample) and only one the mother (this classification excludes step-parents).

The young people were asked a number of questions about the adequacy of communication with their parents. This was based on the parent or step-parent, whoever was considered by the young person to fulfil that role. Because it was based on a number of comments from the interview, the category could include some information from the past and thus some fathers, no longer living in the family home, are included in this analysis. The categories used here are from the interviewer's assessment based on these responses. Their responses were put into three categories: good or adequate, variable, or poor. For the mothers, 35 (57%) seemed to have good or adequate communication, six (10%) variable, and 20 (33%) poor. For the fathers (59), only 26 (44%) were seen as having good or adequate communication, 10 (17%) variable, and 23 (39%) as poor.

The parents were asked at interview to describe the quality of the current communication with the young people. They tended to be more positive in their evaluation. Communication with mothers or stepmothers (in the 81 families to which this applied) was felt to be good by 53 (65%) and adequate by a further 27 (33%). For fathers (72 families) in 33 (46%) of situations it was described as good and in a further 31 (43%) as adequate. The parents were also asked with which of them the young person communicated best and they replied that for 36 (56%) of them it was the mother or stepmother, for 2 (3%) it was the father or stepfather and for the other 26 (41%) it was the same for each parent.

I feel funny about her explaining, because its my own grandparents

The young people were not asked specifically to compare their parents' communication, but were asked a number of questions about communication within the family, leading to a category of whom they communicated with best, shown in Table 2.1. The young people included other family members than just their parents, but this illustrates that, of course, family

Table 2.1. *Family member with whom young person communicates best*

	Number	%
Mother	15	25
Father	3	5
Sibling	12	20
Partner	2	3
Other	2	3
All similar	23	38
No-one	4	7

communication involves more than just the parents; brothers and sisters, grandparents, aunts, uncles and cousins are all involved. While in many families communication was similar with all members, where a family member was best it was most often the mother, or a sibling. Of the 12 who specified siblings, five had deaf siblings. Seven others had deaf siblings and most of these said that communication was similar with all members of the family, perhaps suggesting that the presence of deaf siblings would change communication practices within the family. In general, though, for a substantial number, one in five of the sample, the best communication was with the siblings. Even if they were not deaf, siblings were often felt to have a special sort of understanding with the deaf young people.

> *Shaun learnt Heather some of the hand signs and they communicate sometimes to each other just to...and I don't understand. They talk about me! (laughs)*
> *Mother of Shaun, 21 years, BSL*

> *They've made their own communication up. ( ) We always remind Giles that he should talk to Phillip in the same way as we speak, so it will help him. But Giles doesn't. Giles talks a language which Phillip can understand and Phillip CAN understand! It's unbelievable, they get on like a house on fire.*
> *Father of Phillip, 19 years, SSE*

> *If I can't make her understand I always send her sister, because her sister can. I am a bit of a coward! She can make her understand.*
> *Mother of Bridget, 22 years, BSL*

However, for the young people, the lack of easy communication with grandparents was often the most keenly felt. Sometimes this was a source of frustration and sometimes a sadness, that a relationship, which should be relaxed, was not.

When we go and visit my Gran, my Mum and Gran talk and talk. I understand nothing at all, I want to go out, wander around or go home. They won't sign. I am glad to get home, have tea and dinner and be by myself.
Ivan, 21 years, BSL

My mother helps me understand my grandparents – I feel funny about her explaining because its my own grandparents, I should be able to communicate with them directly.
Rachel, 22 years, BSL

Included in the three who specified the father, is one where the father came from a family with deaf members and could himself sign. In this situation, though, the fact that the father had been brought up in a family where some members were deaf and could sign himself seemed a source of friction.

If she doesn't understand we wait until my father gets home.
Charles, 20 years, BS

My father signs properly like me. My mother doesn't sign. She asks dad what I say. My dad is best. He understands everything I say. () My mum does not like me and my father signing because it makes the dinner go cold. The others talk a lot but if I sign my mother gets angry. She doesn't understand about signing. She has no deaf background but my Dad's family was deaf so he understands.
Charles, 20 years, BSL

PREFERRED LANGUAGE

Until this point, the results have been presented regardless of the preferred language and mode of communication of the young person, or whether or not the parents could sign. As the preferred language of the young people quoted indicates, some of the issues were the same. However, some families did learn to sign and language use within families is considered here. The data are complex, as families differed in their constitution. Some fathers were living in the family home and some were not. The deaf young people could have deaf siblings, hearing siblings or none at all.

Table 2.2 shows the language use of parents and siblings with the deaf young person as perceived by the parents. The category of sign used here is loosely defined. It was not generally possible to ask the parents to specify whether the language used was BSL or whether signs were incorporated into the communication, which could also include speech or gestures. Its

Table 2.2. *The use of language in the families as reported by the parents*

	Parents to young people	Young people to parents	Siblings to young people	Young people to siblings
Oral	35	34	31	31
Oral and gesture	18	18	17	17
Gesture	3	3	5	5
Sign (see text)	25	26	25	25
Writing	1	0	0	0

use then is generous and could imply only the use of few signs, although in some families the use of signs was extensive. It is probably fair to say that in only one family was BSL used to any extent, and this only by the father who had learnt it because of deafness in his own family. As we shall see, the young people were far less likely to describe their parents as using sign language, because they used stricter criteria. However, we felt it relevant to recognise families where the parents spoke of using signs, because of the positive attitude to signing this implied. We had no way of assessing the quality of the signed communication during the interviews with the parents.

However, we were able to distinguish signs from gestures by probing this issue at the interview. 'Signs' implies the use of some of the signs of British Sign Language and were usually learnt at sign language classes or from the young person. Sometimes the signs were demonstrated at the interview by the parents. The term 'gestures' is used when the emphasis in the description was on showing or miming. In the interview, parents did not systematically distinguish between themselves in terms of different language or mode use with the young person. Where there was a difference, the communication of the most competent communicator is given.

As ten of the sample had deaf siblings, it might be felt that this would mean that communication incorporating signs would be most likely to occur with siblings. The fact that this was not the case is because almost always if there was more than one deaf son or daughter in the family, the parents would also acquire some signs.

How did this relate to the young people's preferred language? As the figures are relatively similar across the categories, we shall look only at the language used by the parents, to reduce complexity.

Table 2.3 shows that the situation was relatively clear-cut for those young people who were oral, as the parents were oral with them, a few

Table 2.3. *Young people's preferred language and communication with young people as reported by the parents*

Parent's communication with young people	Young people's preferred language			
	BSL	SSE	Oral	LLS
Oral	5	4	26	0
Oral plus gesture	9	4	4	1
Gesture	0	0	0	3
Sign	16	5	0	4
Writing	1	0	0	0

supplementing the oral communication with gesture. For half of those with limited language skills, the parents were using some signs, and in three situations it was gesture alone, while in one it was speech plus gesture. However, for the young people whose preferred language was BSL, only half the parents used any signs at all, although they were more likely to accompany their speech by gesture than for those young people whose preferred language was oral.

How does this compare with the young persons' perception of the situation? The communication to the young people as perceived by them is shown in Table 2.4. The young people distinguished speech plus finger spelling from other categories. This means that no signs were used. The category of siblings is more complex, for unlike the parents, the young people distinguished communication with different siblings. This was particularly necessary when there were both deaf and hearing siblings.

The young people were far less likely to report the use of signs by their parents; for the mothers this was only 16% (10/61) compared with the parents' report of 30% (25/82). This is largely accounted for by the different definitions employed. With the parents any use of signs counted, while the young people had more rigorous criteria.

Again we need to look at how this related to the young persons' preferred language, and again for convenience we shall look at just one group (see Table 2.5). This shows a similar pattern to that reported by the parents. As one might expect, communication with those young people who were oral was speech, which in three families was accompanied by gesture, but with the BSL users only half the mothers used any signs at all. With the fathers this decreased to 21% (5/24).

Table 2.4. *Communication used with young people, as reported by
young people*

	By mother	By father	By siblings
Speech	40	38	30
Speech plus gesture	7	6	5
Speech plus finger spelling	4	4	4
Speech plus sign	10	8	8
BSL	0	1	0
Writing	0	2	0
Different for different siblings	0	0	8
Not applicable	0	2	6

Table 2.5 *Form of communication used by the mother as reported by
the young person, and young person's preferred language*

	BSL	SSE	Oral
Speech	12	5	23
Speech plus gesture	3	1	3
Speech plus finger spelling	1	3	0
Speech plus sign	8	2	0

CHANGING ATTITUDES TO COMMUNICATION

Working at communication

We have already established that a substantial number of the young people
in the study used BSL or SSE as their preferred means of communication. It
is also clear from the last section that some members of some families also
used signs in their communication with the young deaf person. This is
despite the fact that when the deaf young people were children, all the
emphasis was on the development of speech, and BSL was not considered
as a language. At the time of the first study, communication was seen by
professionals, and consequently parents, as synonymous with speech or
'talk'. The dominant communication philosophy of that time was 'oralism' and none of the parents were even thinking about signing with their
children, let alone actually doing it. Most had been advised not to use any
gestures at all. The advice was uncompromising.

If you want your child to talk in a normal way, you must speak to him
(sic) as you would to any young child, not in an unusual manner. If you
persist in using gesture or pantomime he will not trouble to learn to

talk. He will imitate you and learn that it is easier to get what he wants by gesturing. After that you are going to find it difficult to establish good speech as the means of communication. In order to compete and conform as an adult good speech is essential.   (Ling, 1968)

A child who signs 'Bed me there' instead of saying 'My bed is in there' is leaving out two important words 'is' and 'in' is confusing 'me' with 'my' and puts bed first instead of second. This jumbled way of thinking becomes so ingrained that if he persists with signs, he will have great difficulty in both reading and writing.   (Dale, 1967)

This was reiterated in the advice given to parents in the face-to-face situation by teachers of the deaf.

The teacher who was there then () what has always been very good for Josie and was valuable to me, was she said, 'Don't use too much sign language to Josie, make her lip read, because when you go into the world', which is perfectly true of course, 'very few people can do sign language anyway and if she can lip read she will find communication a lot more easier.
Mother of Josie, 24 years, BSL

Miss N... said they live in a hearing world. She felt that by learning to speak they could communicate which I agree with totally. We didn't encourage him to sign.
Mother of Terry, 22 years, oral

In fact though, many parents dismissed this advice not to gesture and found it impossible to carry out. At the time, 72% of the parents reported using gesture, and of these, 83% felt all right about using it, although 9% disapproved of themselves for gesturing, and a further 8% were ambivalent. For the vast majority of these families the main problem they perceived at that time was around communication, not expressed in terms of the form of communication they should use but simply the issue of how to make themselves understood, and how to understand their own children.

He used to use gesture. There was a constant push for oral communication and yet in the nitty-gritty of it all you used to use a combination of oral and gesture.
Mother of Gavin, 19 years, oral

The earlier study demonstrated the effort that many of the parents put into developing their child's communication, and many still remembered it, now their children are adults. For families of deaf children, the develop-

ment of communication often becomes an end in itself; it becomes the
focus for professional intervention and it becomes the family's, more
particularly the mother's, work.

*Well, our life has revolved around Wayne. I mean he has got an older
brother – eight years – but our life has revolved around Wayne, hasn't
it? It first started off when they came and brought the amplifier; we used
to sit in the front room with him with the earphones on and the
amplifier and the microphone, didn't we? Working at communication.*
Mother of Wayne, 21 years, oral

*What little words you did get were a bonus. We tried to get her to talk, it
was such hard work, a lot of hard work went into one little word. It was
not hopeless. If you didn't use that one little word a lot, it's forgot.*
Mother of Shirley, 22 years, SSE

*Say he wanted a biscuit, he knew where the biscuit tin was and he would
just stand there and go 'ah!'. Well I had to make him make a different
noise to start with and we progressed and I kept saying 'biscuit' and we
progressed where he would say the 'b' and he could never have the
biscuit until he had said the 'b' and when he said 'biscuit' he was never
allowed a biscuit until he said 'biscuit' from then on. And that is how he
went on with everything. And also I spent two hours every day on the
floor with him playing and talking. It was just a two-hour non-stop
break. Just talking and playing, you know.*
Mother of Nigel, 19 years, oral

*Oh yes, then we pinned names on everything. You know 'curtains',
'chair' – these names were everywhere! It was like a museum, 'wall',
'curtains', 'chair' 'table' – we used to carry her around looking at these
and saying the word.*
Mother of Carol, 23 years, oral

One mother, in the later interview, reiterated her earlier feelings concerning the need to talk all the time.

*It's more difficult talking to her. You do get used to it, but even then it's
a bigger strain having her up in the evening than Sharon (her sister). You
have to keep talking to her all the time. It's an effort when you're tired to
be patient and talk.*
Mother of Janet, 6 years (DCF, p. 117–18)

*Mother: (The advice was) just generally to talk to the child as much as
possible, making sure that she could see.*

Father: What you actually did after that was to talk to Janet all the time, no matter what you were doing, getting dressed, washing up, anything, it was talk, talk, talk and you did most of it because I was at work from 9 to 5 and of course that really gave Janet the language she has got today. Talking, talking, talking all the time.

Mother: I used to lift her up when I was tying her shoes and she could see my face and I would have her sitting on the sink when I was washing up so that I could talk to her when I was washing up.

Then I used to have another little session every afternoon with the headphones.

Parents of Janet, 22 years, oral

We ought to have been taught to sign and we ought to have been taught to sign from the word go

So what has happened to these families, and what are the results of all that work on language? Well, 39% (32) of them have learnt to sign, although not all of them sign with their deaf sons and daughters.

As can be seen from Table 2.6, only one parent learnt to sign before their child was school age, and more than half did not start until their child was older than 11 years. Half learnt to sign from their own deaf child and half from classes.

For some of the parents learning to sign came from a straightforward need to communicate with their own children.

Oh yes, I wanted to learn to be helpful to Rachel, you know. () Rachel gets frustrated if you don't know what she's on about. () She used to be trying to talk to us and I'd say, 'I don't know what you mean' and she really was, you know, angry.
Mother of Rachel, 22 years, BSL

We'd be lost without it. Let's put it this way, we have to have sign language to communicate with each other.
Mother of Teresa, 22 years, BSL

Interestingly, nearly a quarter of those who learnt to sign (7/32, 22%) did so, because they needed it to communicate not with their own child but with his or her friends. As their child got older and began bringing home deaf friends, signing became essential in order to enter the social life of their sons and daughters. This mother has learnt to sign but does not use sign language with her daughter, although her daughter signs to her own friends. She explains why she started to learn:

Table 2.6. *Age of child when parents learnt to*
sign

	Number	%
Pre-school (under 5)	1	3
Primary age (5–11)	14	44
Secondary age (12–16)	13	41
Post-school (16+)	4	13

I have always wanted to learn it and when the opportunity came up I
said I would learn it. She has a lot of friends that use sign language and I
would like to be able to communicate with them as well.
Mother of Rosemary, 21 years, oral

I think they should learn sign language. Our children were banned from
using signs in school. Zoe grew up with no sign language. She had to
learn sign language when she was 16. I am learning it now; I've taken the
Stage 1 exam. I'm finding it useful when Zoe's friends come; I am able to
communicate with them a bit.
Mother of Zoe, 19 years, BSL

However, there were one or two young deaf people who did not welcome
their parents signing in this way.

My husband was watching a television programme recently on signing.
When Darren's friends come they sign and my husband thought he
would quite like to learn signing. Darren was horrified. 'We could sign
to your friends then.' 'No it's private, it's for deaf people.' Very
strongly, almost if you can sign then you will know everything about us.
You already know too much about us anyway, but now you'll know
everything. A lot of deaf people feel like that.
Mother of Darren, 22 years, BSL

For families who started out with a commitment to the oral approach with
their children the decision to introduce signing could be very difficult, and
was sometimes made more so by the negative attitude of the authorities.
Some families met with considerable opposition in their attempts to try
and learn sign language. This mother had been committed to the oral
approach when her child was young, but later changed her mind. When
Paula was six years old, her mother said:

I think I use gestures more than I should. I think I shouldn't because
they're not sentences. ( ) I think this puts her in the position of not

watching my lips enough.
Mother of Paula, 6 years (DCF, p. 125)

Later when Paula was 24, her mother talked about this advice.

At the time you are actually very grieved and it sounds sensible at the time. You are living in a normal world, therefore you should communicate in a normal way as everybody else does and it makes it easier for the normal way of going on. It seems reasonable at the time.
Interviewer: When you say 'at the time' it sounds like you've changed.
No it wasn't actually at the time either, because half way through, when Paula was about ten, I realised that there were a lot of things I could not explain properly.
Mother of Paula, 24 years, BSL

She went on to explain that she had enrolled for signing classes but when the school found out they were 'absolutely horrified' to use her own words. She went on to say:

They said I would do a tremendous amount of harm if I pursued this and so I stopped. I mean you do take advice, you have to take advice, and all I can say is I made a disastrous mistake, I should not have listened to them. Until last year they held exactly the same views, very strongly, so it isn't that I happened to be there at the wrong time, it is a very strongly held view that they have and they are wrong.

This mother eventually did learn to sign but not to communicate with her daughter but with her friends.

I went back two years ago (to classes). That wasn't to communicate with Paula – I communicated with her perfectly without signs – it was to communicate with her friends.
Mother of Paula, 24 years, BSL

Advice from professionals carries a lot of weight, especially with a group of parents of deaf children who may not know other parents in a similar position and thus have nothing with which to compare the advice they receive.

Many parents' initial reluctance to use signing was the way in which it seemed an 'either or' choice. The view presented to parents was that if their child learnt to sign they may not speak and this would cut them off from the ordinary world. This struck a chord in most parents.

They said they didn't want you to sign – they objected to signing and I did as well, because you can't communicate with anybody when you are

*out – I mean he started with normal speech. His first word was mother
and it sounded like mother.*
Mother of Nigel, 19 years, oral

*You see we had it explained to us when Christopher was first diagnosed
as being deaf, not to sign to him because it would make him lazy. He
wouldn't speak because they had to put so much effort into speaking
and not so much into signing or pointing because that just makes them
lazy. So that was why we were discouraged.*
Mother of Christopher, 21 years, BSL

*I was absolutely terrified that if she learnt sign language from the word
go, with her being profoundly deaf I felt that once she gets into this sign
language, into the swing of it, it would be her only form of communication. Now, horrible as this sounds, she is in the minority and she has to
go out into the hearing world and everybody is not going to learn sign
language for Isabel, you see. So I felt she must learn to communicate
with hearing people as best she can at their level.*
Mother of Isabel, 21 years, SSE

Like most of the parents who felt positively about signing, Isabel's mother
wanted her child to develop oral skills as far as possible. Later on she
explained how she now felt that Total Communication would have been
'idyllic'. She described herself as being badly informed and felt educators
were 'grovelling in the dark'. To her, the approach seemed to be, 'We will
do this for a bit, see how that works, if it doesn't work we will try
something else'.

*I, in those days, was totally against British Sign Language. But now I
don't feel like that anymore. I feel Total Communication should be
used in all schools for the deaf and I strongly believe that now. Now
Isabel has gone through the system – I really believe all children should
be taught Total Communication.*
Mother of Isabel, 21 years, SSE

Most parents who saw a place for signing did not see this to mean the
neglect or exclusion of speech.

*I thought the most important thing to do was speak, but now I have my
doubts, because I have seen both and I think you have got to have both.*
Mother of Robert, 22 years, BSL

*They were full of advice and I was ignorant. And then when we found
out, that was when we realised that improvements could be made and
we asked for improvements. All the things that we understood. So they*

got equipment to improve their oral teaching. Well, it wasn't getting to the nub of the real problem of the profoundly deaf who needed more communication. They were in no way even going to teach them finger spelling, not even to supplement the oral and that alone is a help. () They wouldn't have any of it. 'Pooh pooh, never do anything like sign language. A low culture, low grading. You never would communicate in the hearing world if you only communicate with the other deaf'. I said 'You have to have both; you are teaching them to speak to the hearing and with the signing they can speak to each other'.
Mother of Helen, 23 years, SSE

One also wonders what attitudes to deaf people are conveyed in a School for the Deaf mentioned in the last quote, where sign language is seen as part of a low culture, a low grading.

While 32 (39%) of parents attempted to learn sign language, 50 (61%) did not. Many of those who did not learn to sign regretted it or later expressed the feeling that it would have been of benefit. For some of these there were feelings of resentment that they had not been introduced to sign earlier.

We ought to have been taught to sign and we ought to have been encouraged to sign from the word go.
Father of Christopher, 21 years, BSL

At another point in the interview the father described how they were discouraged from signing. 'I think it is a damned disgrace.'

We wish we learnt it earlier, to learn sign language right from the word go.
Mother of Jean, 22 years, SSE

I think we should have had signing as well, as a back-up. Definitely, I think we could have used it from day one.
Mother of Melanie, 18 years, BSL

For a few of those who did not learn to sign there was criticism from their offspring. This mother had been committed to an oral approach throughout. When Colin was six years old his mother said:

It's important for him to use language because we want him to be able to speak and communicate with normally hearing people.
Mother of Colin, 6 years (DCF, p. 125)

Later she said how she had tried to do what was best and followed the advice of professionals.

*When you have got a handicapped child you want what is best and you
take advice from professional as to what is best. We thought we were
doing the right thing...But Colin himself would accuse us – he would
say, 'You make life very hard for me because I don't fit in anywhere. I
don't fit into a deaf world and I don't fit into a hearing world.' He
couldn't speak well enough to fit into a hearing world and he couldn't
sign well enough to fit into a deaf world, so life was very hard and he got
very upset and frustrated.*
Mother of Colin, 24 years, BSL

He doesn't use sign language at all. He's never been taught it. He doesn't need it

Even among those who had encouraged speech and whose children had
grown up orally, many saw a place for sign language and were accepting of
sign language for those who preferred it.

*I think you see that she doesn't need to sign and if she can be as close to
the normal patterns of behaviour, speech behaviour and gesture
behaviour, as possible, well, that's all right. But I wouldn't argue
against signing for those people who can't communicate, because they
have got to get through to somebody in some way, otherwise their lives
could be complete isolation and misery.*
Mother of Janet, 22 years, oral

The number who strongly supported oralism, in the sense that they felt
that oralist approaches should be used with all deaf children, was very very
small.

*If you teach them sign language and put them all together, that's how
they speak to each other. If you want them to speak, they've got to be
amongst people who they've got to speak to. He doesn't use sign
language at all. He's never been taught it. He doesn't need it, it was a
deliberate policy not to teach Alistair sign language, so he had to speak.*
Father of Alistair, 21 years, oral

This family are totally against sign language, believing that you have 'to be
cruel to be kind'.

*Yes, there was a phase when our two were still being looked after under
that system (oralism), when the talk came in about sign language. I
think we even went to one of the meetings.. when they were stressing
that we were going to have to bring in the American system of signing*

with speech and actions...By then I think we were convinced that there was nothing to beat forcing them to speak and we may have been indoctrinated but we wouldn't have given in.

Father of David, 20 years, oral

Such views were almost always those of the less deaf children, and those holding such views numbered six or eight from the sample of 82 (7–10%), depending on the strictness of the criteria used. A study of deaf young people (17–20 years) in the late 1970s reported that 39/75 (52%) of parents had positive attitudes to signs, and 35/75 (47%) were negative. One family did not respond (Denmark *et al.*, 1979). It seems clear to us that our research shows a major shift in attitude towards an acceptance of signing among the parents of deaf children who have grown up in the 1970s and 1980s. This of course reflects a general change in attitude and the parents themselves felt that overall society's attitudes to deaf people has changed.

While a change in attitude in our sample took place in the context of an increasing acceptance of sign language in society, it should not be thought that the decisions on communication mode were made easily. Hearing parents of deaf children find themselves in a very difficult situation, and none that we spoke to would have pretended the solution was easy. They were concerned to be able to communicate with their child, but they are also concerned that their child would be able to communicate in the wider family and social group. They wanted their child to grow up and to have friends with whom they could feel relaxed and happy, and they also recognised that few people, in the wider population, can sign.

EARLY COMMUNICATION AND LATER LANGUAGE

In the first interview study reported in *Deaf Children and their Families* it was apparent that, even when the children were young, some of the parents felt more positive about the use of gesture than others, or felt they had no alternative. Furthermore, some children were already manifesting more difficulties in developing spoken language than others. It is important to ask whether these differences persisted, and how they related to later communication. In order to look at this, we shall consider only those 60 children who were three years six months or over at the time of the first interview, so aspects of their communication will be clearer.

Table 2.7 shows that of the sample, 45 (75%) used gesture, while 15 (25%) did not when their children were young. Omitting those with limited language skills from the analysis, we find there is a significant

Table 2.7. *The use of gesture by parents and their feelings about its use*
as related to preferred language of the young people

	BSL	SSE	Oral	LLS
Uses, approves	13	8	6	4
Uses, disapproves	4	2	1	1
Uses, ambivalent	3	0	1	2
Does not use, disapproves	1	0	8	0
Does not use, ambivalent	0	1	4	1

relationship between early use of gesture and later preferred language
($\chi^2 = 18.142$, $p < 0.001$). Those who preferred BSL or SSE were more likely
to have parents who used gesture with them early in their lives than those
who did not. However, if we consider whether or not they approved of
gesture, we do not find a significant relationship with later preferred
language ($\chi^2 = 6.608$, not significant) although there is a significant
relationship if we combine BSL and SSE in the analysis ($\chi^2 = 6.259$,
$p < 0.05$). Thus, if parents approved of gesture early on, their sons and
daughters were more likely to use BSL or SSE as young people, although
this relationship is not as robust as that with actual use of gesture early in
life. To use gesture was to take a step counter to the advice that had been
given. It seems that families took this step if they needed to do this to
communicate, and this was not consequent on their own attitudes to the
use of gesture.

If we now look at the predominant communication, both to the young
person and from the young person, we also find differences with respect to
later preferred language, as shown in Table 2.8. Excluding those with
limited language skills, and combining the categories 'gesture' and 'both'
to give a comparison between speech only or communication involving
gesture, we find a significant relationship with the preferred communication as a child (both receptive and expressive) and later with preferred
language ($\chi^2 = 11.064$, $p < 0.01$). Those children who used and preferred to
receive gesture were more likely as young adults to prefer BSL. Again, a
preference for SSE showed more similarities with the BSL group than the
oral group. It should, however, be noted that there were substantial
proportions of children who were using the spoken word, who later
preferred BSL, and who used gesture, but later were oral.

Table 2.9 shows the language competence of the young person as a child
in terms of their spoken language at that time and their later preferred
language. Excluding those with limited language skills, and comparing
those who used sentences with those who used single words only (both five

Table 2.8. *Preferred communication as child and as young person*

	BSL	SSE	Oral	LLS
As a child, receptive				
Spoken word	3	2	12	0
Gesture	9	3	2	6
Both	9	6	6	2
As a child, expression				
Spoken word	3	2	12	0
Gesture	13	6	5	7
Both	5	3	3	1

words or less and six words or more) we find a significant relationship between early language use and later preferred language ($\chi^2 = 20.818$, $p < 0.001$). As a young child, those who were later oral were more likely to use sentences than users of BSL or SSE. Again, SSE users were more similar to BSL users than to those who became oral. This was examined for the smaller group of those 3.6–4.11 years of age at the first interview, to check that it was not an age effect, but the same result occurred, although the smaller numbers meant that the level of significance was not as high.

Table 2.9 shows up an interesting anomaly, which is not easy to explain. We would expect those who had limited language skills as young children to have poorer language when they were young adults, and this is the case for seven of the eight. However, one was apparently using sentences as a child. A check on this young person's interviews shows this to be correct; he was clearly reported as having 78 words at the time of the first interview when he was three years nine months old. Examples of sentences he used were given, and he could combine two or three words. The later interview with his mother was ambiguous on his language. Overall, her perception of him was of someone with potential who had been let down by the system. However, when he himself was interviewed, the interview had to be abandoned, as he could not respond to the questions. The mother's attitude at this point was different, apologising for his lack of language and also curious as to how we would communicate with him. This situation is discussed further in Chapter 7.

Overall, though, it is clear that children who are likely to grow up to use either BSL or SSE as their preferred language are likely at an early age to show a preference for communication that includes gesture, and are slower at developing spoken communication. This is not a surprising result, and clearly hearing loss will be a major factor here. It is important to note, however, that the parents' approval or disapproval of gesture appears to be of less relevance than the child's own requirements.

Table 2.9. *Language use by N as a child and later preferred language*

	BSL	SSE	Oral	LLS
Sentences	3	1	15	1
Six or more words, not sentences	10	7	4	0
Five words or less	8	3	1	7

CONCLUSION

This chapter may seem to make depressing reading. Even where the young deaf person and their family had established good communication it could still be an effort, particularly in group situations, and the young deaf person often felt excluded from general information within the family and the decision-making process. Often the responsibility for communication lay with one family member, usually the mother or a sibling. In many families the father had poor communication with the young person. Only a minority of the families had had the opportunity to learn sign language and this came very late to most of them. Where families had learnt to sign, it had facilitated communication and most felt they should have been offered information and advice about sign language from the start.

CHAPTER THREE

Experiences of education

Deaf children should have the experience of hearing people so they can communicate, and with deaf people so they can learn about themselves.
Zoe, 19 years, BSL

To deny the chance of contact with other deaf children of similar intellectual level and interests is cruel.
Mother of Christine, 21 years, SSE

Really what you want is normality.
Mother of Paula, 24 years, BSL

The issues of language and communication raised in the last chapter resonate through this one, for they are integral to any discussion of the education of deaf children. The issues are complex. In our sample, the young people differed greatly in terms of language preference and language competence. How best should deaf children be educated? Special school or integrated setting? Using sign language, spoken language, written language or a combination?

There is a vast body of literature on the education of deaf children, but nearly all from the perspective of the educationalists and other involved professionals. All too often the topic is discussed at a theoretical level far removed from the practical everyday experiences of its consumers – young deaf people and their families. The issues have been debated for many years by educationalists, by psychologists and by the Deaf community itself. It is an area in which opinions tend to be polarised and feelings run high. Each group has its own frame of reference and each its own criteria

Table 3.1. *Type of school attended at the various stages*

	Infant		Junior		Secondary	
	Number	%	Number	%	Number	%
School for the deaf	47	58	49	60	45	55
PHU	24	30	20	25	23	28
Mainstream	9	11	11	14	11	13
Other special school	1	1	1	1	3	4
Total[a]	81		81		82	

Note: [a] For a child who was fostered, clear information about school placement was not available for the infant and junior stage.

for judging success. A missing element in the discussion has been the view of young deaf people and their families. This chapter may go a little way towards putting that perspective forward and redressing the balance.

Overall, we were struck by the very thoughtful and considered way in which the families and young people expressed their opinions. For the most part, they had an appreciation of both sides of the major educational debates. They had little time for dogma. They spoke from personal experience and only rarely with bitterness. We invited both the parents and the young people to talk about their own specific experiences and offer their opinions on issues under general debate; often these experiences informed opinions in a compelling way.

In order to provide a context for the discussion we look first at the settings in which these young deaf people experienced their education. The schools attended by the young people at various stages of their school career are shown in Table 3.1. Where this changed during the period of a particular stage, the final placement is indicated.

As can be seen from Table 3.1, at any one time most of the sample were in schools for the deaf. However, the relative consistency of the figures may give a false impression in terms of consistency of placement for individual children. In fact, many of the sample experienced changes in type of placement at transition points in their school career. Only 37 (46%) were placed in the same type of provision for the whole of their school careers. Seven attended partially hearing units throughout, while a further six at junior and secondary school only. Five were integrated throughout, with four being integrated through junior and secondary schools. Only 25 attended schools of the deaf throughout, and a further six attended schools for the deaf through junior and secondary stages only. Of those 25 attending schools for the deaf throughout, eight boarded throughout their school career and six were non-boarders throughout. The others had a pattern of boarding and non-boarding, the majority (8/11) boarding at secondary school only.

DIFFERENT EDUCATIONAL SETTINGS

Hearing and deaf don't mix

We were all friends from the same village

While all educational settings were endorsed by some and rejected by others based on their own experiences, overall those who had attended schools for the deaf tended to be happiest with the education they had received.

> *Interviewer: what was your favourite school?*
> *B... (special school), as there were more people and lots of different subjects. It was very strict but that did not bother me. It was close, like a family.*
> *Isabel, 21 years, SSE*

> *I liked the E... School because everyone was deaf. When I went to the Unit it was mixed. I found it very confusing with the hearing children. The E... School was best for learning and for friends.*
> *Sam, 18 years, BSL*

But while the two young people quoted above found the level of education at their special school good, where there were criticisms of special education, it usually concerned the low standards and expectations.

> *Upper school was rubbish. It was all baby talk. I was not happy there. The teachers were lazy. They didn't make us work hard. They didn't teach us enough language.*
> *Rachel, 22 years, BSL*

This issue of low attainments was a recurring theme for all forms of educational provision, and one to which we shall return.

Others complained that their school for the deaf had failed to prepare them for the hearing world, either by not alerting them to the problems or by minimising the difficulties they would face.

It's all right for deaf children to go to deaf schools but they need to know what hearing people are like – it was a shock for me when I went to college.
Brenda, 21 years, SSE

M... school pushed us to have high expectations of ourselves. It was a real shock when we left and had to pull ourselves down.
Deborah, 20 years, oral

When I left school I was lost. At M.. school I was with deaf people all the time. Now I am in the world with hearing people all the time. It's like having to start all over again.
Veronica, 21 years, SSE

Partially hearing units seem, in theory, to offer the best of both worlds – the company of other deaf children and access to the hearing world. However, there were limitations, both because of the small numbers and the degree of integration that took place.

I was happiest at P... Unit. I could understand best of all. I had a few deaf friends and I kept in the small oral class. It was difficult to break out of the group, though.
Fiona, 22 years, SSE

At B... Unit they were very helpful all the time. Some people had the same problems as me, others more, others different problems with speech and so on. I stayed in the same group, I was happy with them, I was not abused, I could understand everything, I could follow all the time.
Mark, 22 years, oral

Several, however, complained of fighting and teasing within units settings.

When deaf children go to a hearing school the hearing tease them and they end up fighting.
Ivan, 21 years, BSL

Hearing and deaf don't mix. When they are together at playtimes and mealtimes they fight all the time.
Gary, 21 years, oral

The approach that brought forth the most emotive responses was integration. Some enjoyed this situation, for the relationships they formed and for the high level of education. Even the difficult times were seen by some as a good preparation for life outside school.

The school always expected the best, encouraged you and kept you going to do your best.
David, 20 years, oral

Junior School was very protective – everyone was friendly and I wasn't aware of any horrible children. The secondary school helped me grow up and develop as a person – being put in with horrible children who were not as understanding and sympathetic as the junior school pupils. I think I enjoyed the educational side, the teaching, of the sixth form. I had a choice of subjects as I had exams to do.
Ruth, 19 years, oral

I was happiest at H... we were all friends from the same village. We used to play at school and after school when we got home. My friends always helped if I had problems. Then I went to ... (Unit) because I needed extra help. The children there were sometimes spiteful.
Jonathan, 22 years, oral

This contrast was reversed, however, for others. Mark, who above commented favourably on the Unit he attended, said this about integration:

My whole time at D... was wasted. In my reports I was always last, because everyone else could hear and their brain developed, but not me. I tried to lip read but it didn't go in, it didn't stay there. I couldn't lip read very well. The law changed (reference to corporal punishment) but in that school they gave it to you and I never knew what for. Mr J... called me over, everyone was standing by the window – and he gave me four. I can remember how painful it was, but not why. After school everyone was running after me, kicking me.
Interviewer: Did your mother know?
Yes, but she couldn't do anything about it.
Mark, 22 years, oral

There were also suggestions that in integrated settings some deaf pupils could develop lower self esteem.

Some of my friends went to hearing schools – they feel they are lower than the hearing children.
Nicky, 21 years, SSE

VIEWS ON EDUCATIONAL PLACEMENT

The young people

The hearing must understand the deaf and the deaf must understand the hearing

Janet: Based on my experience, you need deaf and hearing schooling to give you a balance in life. You need to be part of the deaf world and the hearing world. I would send it (a deaf child) to a hearing primary school, and, I don't know, maybe then a Unit. It is very hard to decide.

Andrew: I'm profoundly deaf. Talking is all right but I can't understand hearing people – they go too fast for me. I need to go to a deaf school and learn more sign and English before I leave...Hearing people talk quickly behind people's backs. It's better to go to a deaf school than watching lips all the time. Hearing people talk fast and I can't follow.

Tina: I agree. The Partially Hearing Unit is not very good – I did not learn much. Lip reading is all I did most of the time to understand what people were saying.

Jeremy: When I was 3–7, I went to morning classes in a Unit and in the afternoon ordinary classes...I'm split between the two ideas. It depends on personal confidence. There should be discussion between the deaf child, parents and social worker. If the child is confident enough, it should be their choice. My preference is that they go to normal school. They've got to be self-confident. If someone calls me names, usually thump them or call back and they leave me alone.

Group leader: But what about schools for people as deaf as Andrew? He said his ideal education would be in a school for the deaf.

Jeremy: The parents, social workers and child should all choose together – it should be their choice. That sort of school might not be the best for someone as deaf as Andrew. I think that type of school is too protective. When I left my school I was more confident than I would have been if I had left a school for the deaf. Leaving a school for the deaf is a bit like coming out of a shell into the big wide world, you're not quite sure what to expect – such as people's attitudes to you and vice versa.

(From a group discussion with deaf young people interviewed for the research)

The previous section gives some impression of the widely differing experiences and views of the young people. What, then, did they them-

Table 3.2. *The young people's view of the*
best school setting for deaf pupils

	Number	%
School for the deaf	19	34
Integration	4	7
Integration (modified)	9	16
PHU	5	9
Depends (hearing loss, 13; personality, 4; age, 2)	19	34

selves feel was the best way to educate deaf children? In the discussion
reported above, many of the points, central to the debate on educational
placement, were raised. This conversation brings out clearly the issues
involved – the need for the curriculum to be delivered in a language which
is accessible, the need to learn about the hearing world and the need to
learn about the deaf world.

Towards the end of their individual interviews the young people were
asked what they felt to be the best provision for deaf pupils. Two of them
said they did not know and three of them did not answer the question. The
responses of the 56 who did answer, are given in Table 3.2. The greatest
proportion, one-third, favoured schools for the deaf.

> *It's better that all deaf people are together. It's better for talking. Before,*
> *I was with hearing people and I didn't understand.*
> Gavin, 19 years, oral

> *Deaf children should be in deaf schools. In deaf schools they can give*
> *extra time for language. In hearing schools it's so hard to communicate*
> *that deaf children give up. I am not sure about Units. Maybe a Unit is*
> *sometimes where the deaf try to be like hearing people.*
> Isabel, 21 years, SSE

Nearly a quarter were in favour of integration of some sort, for the
experience it gave of the hearing world.

> *They've got to be integrated – if signers are all together they have no*
> *experience of the real world like normal kids.*
> David, 20 years, oral

It is interesting, however, that many of them who favoured integration
rejected the current practice of individual integration and made different
proposals. It was an indication of how great the concern with education
was among the deaf young people that so many of their responses went

beyond currently available options to propose a system that was more radical.

> *There should be speech and signing. Not Units but 100 deaf and 600 hearing.*
> Paula, 24 years, BSL

> *There needs to be more interest in integrating schools – learning from one another...there shouldn't be one deaf pupil on their own in a class of hearing pupils but four or five in each class. I know the feeling of being on my own – my tension and frustration. If you are with other deaf pupils, there is a natural bond.*
> Phillip, 19 years, SSE

> *They should go to a hearing school but with lots of deaf pupils. It should be a mixed class, deaf and hearing.*
> Darren, 22 years, BSL

Five of the group saw advantages in Units. Interestingly here the consequences were not only seen as for the deaf pupils but also for the hearing.

> *Units, because the hearing must understand the deaf and the deaf need to understand the hearing.*
> Nigel, 19 years, oral

However, a significant number (19, 34%) did not see the issue as clear-cut and felt it depended on various factors – personality, hearing loss or stage of schooling.

> *Mainstream for me was OK. I was confident, but if I'd been a shy person it would probably have been no good. It depends on the child's personality.*
> Jeremy, 20 years, oral

A further interesting proposal was that children should be exposed to different forms of education at different stages in the career. While only two young people made this proposal it was interesting, because it is the reverse of that usually practised, where children attend local schools when they are young and then go on to special settings. There the suggestion was that they should, at primary age, attend special schools to become confident and establish their own identity, and then at secondary stage go on to integrated settings. At this age they needed to learn about the hearing world, they needed a wider range of social contacts. This suggestion may also reflect the fact that, for many of them, the level of education they had received in special secondary school had been very low. This idea was also

Table 3.3. *Secondary school placement and views on the educational placement of deaf children*

	School attended		
Recommended placement	School for deaf	Integration	PHU
School for deaf	15	0	4
Integration	1	2	1
Integration modified	3	0	6
PHU	1	2	2
Depends	8	7	4
Total	28	11	17

reiterated and reinforced in one of the group discussion, with the young people, where it was the consensus view.

> *Paula: From the age of five to ten years I was in a school for the deaf. If hearing children are mixed together with deaf children it is easy to get confused. The hearing children can follow what is going on, the deaf children just sit there, sort of nodding and are not really learning anything. So I think from the age of five until ten it should be a school for the deaf only. After that it does not matter so much; when you are older integration helps to develop confidence for the future, for life with hearing people. I think if you are only with other deaf pupils at secondary school, how would you cope when you left school?*
> *Phillip: Yes, I think at that age (5–10) it should be only deaf children with no hearing children. It should be only signing and no speaking. After ten years old you need to be with hearing pupils as well, to learn to talk. If you mix at secondary school you will learn to speak and be able to use both (speech and sign). If you are only with deaf people all the time, then when you are older you will only be able to make friends with deaf people.*
> *(From a group discussion, with young people interviewed for the research)*

One consideration in this discussion was the extent to which their feelings about provision related to their own experiences of education. Table 3.3 shows their placement at secondary stage and their views on placement. Over half attending schools for the deaf saw them as the preferred means of education for deaf children (15/28, 54%). Most of those attending mainstream settings felt that placement should depend on various factors (7/11, 64%), while only two of the eleven favoured integration. Of those attending partially hearing units, the majority were in favour of some form

Table 3.4. *Parents' views on integration*

	Number	%
Disapprove	28	35
Approve	10	12
Complex	43	53

of integration, but most looked for modifications to the conventional system (6/17, 35%). Only two preferred PHUs, and one integration on the conventional model.

The parents

Father: I think education has changed for the worse. It's gone downhill. I think integration is stupid

Mother: I think it is good

In discussion with the parents, rather than asking them what type of education they felt would be best they were asked more specifically for their views on integration. The introduction of policies of integration in some Local Education Authority areas during the period of the research meant that this was a critical issue for many of them. Their responses are shown in Table 3.4.

The answers they gave clearly indicated the complexity of this issue for parents. It was the major issue on which husbands and wives did not always agree with each other, as the quote which heads this section demonstrates. (Issues around the coding of such responses are discussed in Appendix III.) There was a real dilemma.

If I had been offered normal education for my children when they were young I would have jumped at it, because the thing most parents want is to think there isn't a problem and that they can fit into normal goings on. Really what you want is normality. () I think for Paula, if she'd gone to a normal school, it would have been totally disastrous and speaking as a teacher I have seen far too many children with special needs deprived in main-school education and I have had to teach some of them and I think it is a con put onto parents. If someone had come along to me and said, 'Yes deaf children can manage perfectly well in normal school', I would not have been aware, and it would have taken years to

become aware, of the problems that was going to mean for them in the future. All sorts of things! () No I think you need schools for the deaf up to a certain age. You need to give the basics in schools for the deaf and here I am not talking as a parent, I am talking as a teacher.
Mother of Paula, 24 years, BSL

Only 10 (12%) of the families in interviews gave their unqualified approval for placing deaf children in mainstream schools. The reasons were as often social as educational.

I think it is a good idea. James used to come home on a Friday night, and he was lost because all his friends were at school. There was no-one here apart from his sisters. He didn't have a friendship. I think he would have got on far better in an integrated school. Mixing with people would help. He hadn't mixed with a lot of people until he started work.
Mother of James, 20 years, BSL

Yes (integration) is a much better idea, because if you see children in deaf schools they don't attempt to speak, they use sign language all the time. If you teach them sign language and put them all together, that's how they'll speak to each other. If you want them to speak, they've got to be amongst people who they've got to speak to.
Father of Alistair, 20 years, oral

See, the thing is, when they are away from home and they are not going to a local school they have no local friends. Really, they are isolated, aren't they? You make your friends at school, don't you, and if you're not at the local school then you haven't got any local friends.
Mother of Robert, 22 years, oral

Approximately one-third (28) of the families completely disapproved of integration, often because the current organisation of ordinary schools or class size seemed prohibitive.

I don't think it has a cat in hell's chance of working as it's supposed to. It would never be practical to have profoundly deaf children in an ordinary local comprehensive. Even if you have a system where they can be educated in a normal school, to deny her the chance of contact with other deaf children of a similar intellectual level and interests is cruel.
Mother of Christine, 21 years, SSE

I don't think it could possibly work without a lot of support and a lot of one-to-one tuition. They've got to learn to communicate before they can learn anything. I know from Nicky's experience at B... College she

couldn't cope with an ordinary classroom situation without individual help.
Mother of Nicky, 21 years, SSE

At the Royal School for the Deaf they have got one teacher to about six or seven pupils and they have got earphones, you know, plugged into one microphone. You know all the equipment – they haven't got it in normal schools, anyway. So she wouldn't have got any education – she would have been stuck in at the back of the class, you know, not doing anything.
Mother of Rachel, 22 years, BSL

It is good as regards mixing and playing and the talking part of it, as you might say, but would they be able to keep up with education? Because, I mean, a teacher couldn't wait for them to catch up with the other 30 or 40 going like the clappers, could she?
Father of Wayne, 21 years, oral

Father: I think education has changed for the worse. It's gone downhill. I think integration is stupid.
Mother: I think it is good.
Father: I don't think you can possibly teach in an integrated school.
Mother: You can.
Father: You can't, because in an integrated class there are too many pupils. The teacher can't afford the time to concentrate on the one that is falling behind. The teacher hasn't got the time. The tendency is to ignore the ones that are behind. It should be the other way round.
Mother and Father of Jenny, 19 years, SSE

However, for over half the parents the issue was more complex and they did not feel able to give straight approval or disapproval. A number (9, 11%) suggested that integration could work but there were major resource implications that currently were not being met.

I've got a lot of sympathy for integrating, because I think it has social values, but if you are going to integrate children then the cost of integration is going to be extremely high and if they must integrate then they must pay for it. And that means providing specialist teachers. It means providing support for teachers who teach the hearing children, so that they know what the problem is. And it needs special equipment, special arrangements, and it needs a specialist who knows what sorts of arrangements need to be made for children with different disabilities, because the arrangements for a child who can't see very well must be different from a child who can't hear very well. To make it simplistic

and say either to integrate or not integrate – really it appears to me there is a problem there.
Father of Janet, 22 years, oral

I think it should have more back-up if it is going to happen. As the system is – no, I am totally against it. I have seen kids being miserable in a playground of all hearing kids and two little deaf kids who are like pinned together.
Mother of Paula, 24 years, BSL

For some (24, 30%) successful integration depended on the level of the child's hearing loss.

For someone with Ruth's level of hearing loss – ideal – given the school that she went to. () Had her hearing loss been any greater I would have said that she would have needed a lot more support.
Mother of Ruth, 19 years, oral

I don't honestly think that a profoundly deaf child would gain anything from a Partially Hearing Unit. Integration is not the be all and end all. They have to be educated in the best...I think those kids...if they are profoundly deaf, would sit nodding their heads or whatever all day long, and probably take in very little.
Mother of Isabel, 21 years, SSE

I think that it is good. Not like Matthew, no...not with the deafness he's got. For a partially hearing child...I do definitely!
Mother of Matthew, 21 years, LLS

Well, possibly for a not quite so profoundly deaf child it might have been better, but for Josie, because she has a dreadful hearing loss, I wouldn't have been happy at all.
Mother of Josie, 24 years, BSL

Parents' and young people's views compared

The questions asked of parents and young people were slightly different so the comparison is not straightforward. However, Table 3.5 shows the comparison between the parents and their sons and daughters for the 56 families where these data were available. Because of the number of parents who said it depends, the comparisons are difficult to make, except to say that if the parent approved of integration it did not necessarily follow that the young person did. However, where the parent disapproved, there was no instance of the young person advocating integration without some

Table 3.5. *Comparison of young people's and parents' view of educational placement*

	Parents' view on integration		
	Approve	Disapprove	Depends
Young person's view on ideal placement			
School for Deaf	2	9	8
Integration	1	0	3
Integration modified	0	2	7
PHU	1	1	3
Depends	2	8	7

modification, and the young people were most likely to recommend schools for the deaf.

SIGN LANGUAGE AND EDUCATION

My teachers told me signing was not good for you

The view of both the young people and their parents on where deaf children should be educated was often influenced by their attitude to the role of sign language in the education of deaf children. As was discussed in Chapter 1, a major controversy in the education of deaf children concerns the language that should be used in schools. The young people in the sample started school at a time when oralism was the main way of educating deaf children, whether they attended special school or a Unit or were integrated into a mainstream school. However, during the period of the research, attitudes to sign language mellowed and some schools actively endorsed signing while others became more tolerant of its use around the school. Some schools did and still do enforce oral approaches.

We were therefore interested to find out the extent to which the young people had been exposed to signing and allowed to sign during their education. The answers of the three (from the young people's interviews) who were mainstreamed throughout their school career are included in the category of those forbidden to sign. Thirteen did not answer the question and the responses of the remaining 48 are given in Table 3.6.

It emerges that only one-quarter of the sample were allowed or encouraged to sign at school and over one-third were forbidden. The 18 (38%) for whom it varied probably reflect the changing attitude and will

Table 3.6. *Experiences of the use of signs at school*

	Number	%
Forbidden	18	38
Allowed	3	6
Encouraged	9	19
Varied throughout school career	18	38

have started in oral education but later been in a situation more tolerant of sign language.

Of course, the issues of school placement and language use are bound up together, though not inevitably so. Although usually oral approaches are more likely in integrated settings and sign language approaches in special settings, the alternatives are possible and exist. Some deaf children in mainstream settings have sign language support. One of the disturbing things about the interviews was not simply the revelations in terms of policy on sign language but the punishments that could be meted out to those caught signing contrary to regulations. Some special schools were and remain exclusively oral, imposing punishments on pupils who did not conform. The following quotes are all from young people who attended special schools for deaf pupils.

If you were caught by the same person three times, you had to stand outside the classroom. If it was more than three times, then they said they would send you to...(a school for children with learning difficulties).
Gary, 20 years, oral

They would slap your hand. They would say, 'Use grown-up talk'.
Gavin, 19 years, oral

I couldn't talk, but I wasn't allowed to sign to the teacher to ask a question. I was hit with a ruler.
Paula, 24 years, BSL

There was a chart of the whole school and bad speech marks were put on the chart to embarrass you. They made a big thing of it. They gave prizes for good speech.
Deborah, 20 years, oral

At B... School, you got your hands slapped. You had to fold your arms and speak. We tried to sign under the desk.
Christopher, 21 years, BSL

My school was oral. The teachers told me signing was not good for you. It wouldn't help communication with hearing people so you must learn to speak. Those with deaf parents formed themselves into a group to sign in private. They used to get 'bad speech marks', lines, and as a punishment they had to stand in the corner or they got a detention.
Veronica, 21 years, SSE

But there were a lot of people at school who relied on sign language anyway, because it was their first language and they got bad speech marks every day for doing it.
Michael, 20 years, oral

In the last two quotes, a group of children are described who came from families where the mother and father were deaf, and sign language was the language they used at home, yet they were punished for using it at school. Such punishment for using one's mother tongue would not have been tolerated with hearing children from minority ethnic groups whose home language was not English.

While the school ideology may have been oral, the pupils themselves could sometimes have a different set of priorities and attitudes, as suggested from this young woman who attended an oral school (one of those referred to above).

At school people rejected me, because I could speak well and got on well with all the teachers. I approached a deaf girl (from a deaf family) I knew and asked her to teach me to sign.
Deborah, 20 years, oral

When asked about the use of sign language in education, of the 51 who were able to answer the question, 20 (39%) favoured approaches that utilise signing, 23 (45%) suggested that it depended on the circumstances and only eight (16%) favoured totally oral approaches. The most passionate endorsements for signing came from those who had attended an oral setting but had great difficulty with speech.

To force people to be oral is a waste of time. Profoundly deaf people like me need signs as well as speech but they (teachers) don't believe that.
Veronica, 21 years, SSE

Signing is good in schools. If you sign you understand and save time. If children speak to the teacher, the teacher doesn't understand. If the children sign to the teacher it saves time, otherwise the teacher makes the child write on the blackboard. I had to do this.
Christopher, 21 years, BSL

As with their views on integration, however, the responses of the young people were mostly moderate rather than extreme, the greatest proportion of them suggesting that there was no single approach that was suitable for all.

> *I think sign language is suitable for deaf people who can't talk, but not for those who can, otherwise they won't learn to talk properly.*
> *Amanda, 20 years, SSE*

DECISIONS CONCERNING SCHOOL PLACEMENT

The parents' role

Probably we did have a role but no-one told us

Given the controversial issues involved, to what extent did the parents feel they had a say in the education their children received? Many of the families felt that they had no choice but to send their children to the schools recommended by their local education authority advisers. In fact, when asked if they had played any part in selecting a school for their children at any stage, the majority of parents (45, 55%) said that they had not. However, 16 of the families had played an active part in choosing infant schools for their children, 15 had chosen at junior school stage and 22 had chosen at secondary stage.

At the primary stage, parents were tending to make choices based on limited knowledge – they knew their children well but they knew very little about the educational choices available to them. Some parents believed that they had no choice and simply followed the advice of professional advisers.

> *We got no choice and that was it! Probably we did have a choice but nobody ever told us. It was B or D.*
> *Mother of Teresa, 22 years, BSL*

Some parents chose not to send their children to special primary schools, preferring them to attend mainstream schools.

> *I wanted to stretch her in a normal class, but they said it would be too much for her and she should start with the Unit first. We didn't agree, so that's when they said that OK we'll put her in this reception class and if she couldn't cope in there by Christmas they wouldn't ask me, they would just take her out and put her in the Unit.*
> *Mother of Jane, 20 years, oral*

The children in this area had to go to K... The authority would only allow them to come home at half-term...We were automatically required to go and look at it (D... School). We felt we would prefer the route of normal schooling.
Father of John, 22 years, oral

Quite often when parents did exercise choice it was for their children NOT to go to a particular school – so they were reacting to negative feelings about the choices on offer rather than actively selecting schools that they preferred. Often too their choices were not based on educational considerations but on emotional ones. This is understandable insofar as the situations being presented were often quite alien to them and totally outside their normal frame of reference. Particularly in the early stages of education the issue of boarding was a real dilemma. The idea of a two-year-old child being educated in a boarding school was something outside their experience. Some accepted it reluctantly, while others just refused.

If Ray was hearing I wouldn't have him board anywhere, but we didn't have any choice.
Mother of Ray, 21 years, oral

We wanted what was best for Nicholas. They offered to put him in a school where he had to go away. He had to go away for the week and come home at weekends. No way was we going to allow that. We would have let him go if it was for his own benefit but we were losing a member of the family. He would have become a complete stranger, because you could not help him. It was left to other people. So, in the end it got to the local councillor with letters to the education authority and oh! I can't remember how many was involved, we had quite a fight on our hands, it wasn't very nice. The outcome was... (a PHU), with a fight. He had to set out early; he had to have a taxi. We were able to help him with his school work and... did everything for him. He really came on in leaps and bounds.
Mother of Nicholas, 24 years, oral

At secondary level more parents were selecting their child's school and also the bases upon which their choices were being made had changed. Parents knew more about their child, more about deafness and more about the educational system as it existed for deaf children.

Over the years we were getting more involved with the deaf children, we saw them going out to the different schools and then we saw them coming back and we were not impressed with it. So we started talking

ourselves a little bit and decided that we didn't want Christopher to be brilliant at running or brilliant at swimming. We didn't want him to be clever at mime and drama and that sort of thing and we didn't particularly want him to be a brilliant artist, because we knew that Christopher had got to take part in what we call the 'real' world. He has got to go out and earn a living and probably, hopefully, marry and support a family. So that is what decided us in the end to send him to a school where they specialised in good speech development. It was very hard, though, making the choice.
Mother of Christopher, 21 years, BSL

So we went all around – did our homework and we found a school at S..., the W... school and we set up there. It was the best we could find. It wasn't perfect but it was the best we could find. We were impressed with the headmaster...his attitude...he was really good; what he wanted to do and what he was going to do with the children and how they would be integrated with the hearing for part of the day. And so we had to go to the authorities and be interviewed and it was a real tussle but my husband was very good at handling that. He did his homework very well and he finally persuaded the powers that be to let him go to the W... school.
Mother of Colin, 24 years, BSL

But as the last quote shows, influencing decisions can be difficult, particularly if a parent felt, as this one did, that 'I have not got that kind of vocabulary' when she questioned decisions that were being made about her own child's future placement.

And you get all this...because he is the professional and I am the fussy mum. You get all this business about, you know; and they blind you with science, you know; because you know he could beat me any day in an argument, because I have just not got that kind of vocabulary. But, you know, you chip away at it, you know.
Mother of Veronica, 21 years, SSE

The significance of this should not be underestimated, as many parents even years later are still reflecting upon the decisions that have been made and wondering if they were the right ones.

And even now we find ourselves saying, 'Well, if she had gone to A instead of B, it would have been marvellous'. We know parents whose children have gone to C and that seems to be marvellous and I find myself thinking if Carol had not gone to B she might have done much

Table 3.7. *The relationship between functional hearing loss and school placement*

	Profoundly deaf	Severely deaf	Moderately deaf	Partially hearing
School for the deaf	22	18	5	0
PHU	7	8	6	2
Integration	0	4	1	6
Other special school	2	0	1	0

better, but she might not have been. How do you know? And you can never go back and do the other thing, it's very sad.
Mother of Carol, 23 years, oral

The influence of the local authority

As might be expected, in general the children with the greater functional hearing loss were likely to attend schools for the deaf. Of the 31 assessed as profoundly deaf, 25 were in schools for the deaf at the infant stage, 29 at the junior stage and 22 at the secondary stage. The pattern is less clear for the milder losses. Of those 21 who were moderately deaf or partially hearing, 16 were in mainstream or PHU at the infant stage, 16 at the junior and 15 at the secondary stage. The way in which hearing loss did not directly reflect school placement is shown in Table 3.7, which shows the relationship between hearing loss and placement at the secondary stage.

Therefore, decisions on placement did not consistently reflect hearing loss or specifically educational factors. Local authorities varied themselves in policy on particular placement issues. We give just three examples. (We have had to use the local authority at the time of the first study for this. There may thus be minor errors, but we have no reason to feel they affect the figures significantly.)

The age of starting full-time education varied from authority to authority. In one area, eight of the 21 children (38%) started at school full time before they were three years old, but in the other four authorities very few started at this early age (0/9, 1/9, 1/18, and 3/24). Communication philosophy also varied. At the infant stage the percentage of children placed in schools with an oral philosophy varied from 89% (16/18) to 54% (12/22). The actual type of placement used also differed. Table 3.8 shows the school placement at secondary stage by authority. We have chosen secondary, as this is the most recent, so these placements were mostly in the last ten years. The chances of being in a school for the deaf varied from

Table 3.8. *School placement by local authority*

	Authority				
	A	B	C	D	E
School for deaf, non boarding	6	2	0	0	4
School for deaf, boarding	10	8	5	6	4
Integration	1	4	2	1	3
PHU	7	4	2	1	9

40% (8/20) to 75% (6/8), an integrated setting from 4% (1/24) to 22% (4/18) and for PHUs it was 13% (1/8) to 45% (9/20). This decision depended largely on the policy of the particular local authority.

ASPECTS OF SCHOOL LIFE

I'll never forget it when she went off that day

For all parents, when their child starts school, it is a major event, but with a deaf child maybe particularly so. In parent interviews we began by asking parents to pick up their thoughts where the first interviews had left them – at the beginning of formal education. This mother remembered her daughter's first day at school as if it had been yesterday.

At the time she didn't have enough language, obviously, for me to explain what school was, or...I stuck her in this taxi with this strange man, clutching a bag and she survived, you know, and then, eventually she realised that she came back home. That must have been quite traumatic. I don't think it was very honourable. I think we could have thought about it. Had we had the money we would probably have had other arrangements but we were pretty hard up.
Mother of Ruth, 19 years, oral

It is probably not surprising that the memory is a vivid one, as starting school is quite an event in the lives of most parents and their children. As the quote showed, this little girl, like many deaf children of her age, did not have the language skills to understand her mother's explanations about starting school. Parents of hearing children usually take for granted the possibility of talking about exciting, confusing and painful events with their children well before they take place; for the most part parents of deaf children have to depend on alternative means. Often the parents of deaf

Table 3.9. *Age of starting school (cumulative data)*

	Number	%
Before three years	13	16
Before four years	50	62
Before five years	70	86
At five years	81	100

children recognised that their children, as a consequence of this, were ill-prepared for experiences in their young lives. Another quote underlines this.

She went to S... special school when she was three. Full time. It was a horrible day. Pushed her into the car, was unable to explain at that age where she was going. Her little face! I'll never forget it when she went off that day. It was an awful day. It was a full-time nursery.
Mother of Amy, 19 years, BSL

A second aspect of the experience, marking it out as different from the usual, is the early age at which the children described above and many deaf children even now enter full-time schooling. As can be seen from Table 3.9, nearly two-thirds of the children in the study had started school full time before their fourth birthday. Thirteen (16%) had started before their third birthday and only 11 started at the most usual age of five years.

Perhaps because of their early start in formal schooling, only around one-third of the children had attended local playgroups or mother–toddler groups. Whilst acknowledging that such voluntary groups are more widespread now, than they were when the children in our study were young, it would seem that these opportunities to establish local friendships were reduced at a time when parents would have most valued them, both for themselves and for their children.

The quotes above highlight a further feature of the education of deaf children, that being the need to travel to school in provided transport. Special schools were unlikely to be within walking distance, as most counties had only one special school for the Deaf and a handful of Units for partially hearing children. One consequence of attending such a school was that taxis or minibuses were used to transport children to them, if the school was reasonably close and within the same county. This could mean a long and exhausting working day for the child, as these quotes imply.

Well, she would come back, you see, absolutely exhausted and would kneel down by the table and put her head on it and go to sleep.
Father of Ruth, 19 years, oral

They have a long day, because the taxi used to come for them soon after eight in the morning and it was nearly five when they came home.
Mother of David, 20 years, oral

I didn't really want to leave him but I knew I had got to

At the time of the study, starting school could also involve going away from home. If the school was outside the county in which the family lived it was more likely that the child would be required to board at school. As can be seen from Table 3.9, 13 of the children (16%) were boarding at infant level, some of them starting as young as three years old. The figure of 16% at infant stage seems very high in the current climate, as attitudes have changed. It would now only be in very exceptional circumstances that a child under five would board, and certainly in the first book the comments of many of the parents of children who did board indicated what a wrench this was. For many the memory remained clear.

She was at D... all the time. It was heart-breaking. We were 60 miles away. She was only three years old. At first she was only allowed home alternate weekends, because they thought that every weekend was unsettling. It was awful and the journey was terrible getting her home. Sunday was ruined, because she didn't want to go back. She went through phases. The first year or so she seemed to accept what went on. I am sure she felt rejected, but the staff there were marvellous in trying to replace the care. They were good, I can't fault them. It's just the heartlessness of a virtual baby being away from home. She cried on Sundays. She didn't want to go back. Not so much the first year, but as she got older she would refuse to go and she would have tantrums. It was absolute agony sometimes. There was no other way she was going to be educated.
Mother of Nicky, 21 years, SSE

Well, the worst part was him starting school...well, it was just the leaving him there and the having to leave him, like. It was that hard.
Mother of Ivan, 21 years, BSL

Although the impact of boarding may have been greatest for children at the youngest ages, the impact of boarding was important throughout. The proportion who attended a boarding school for deaf children, at each stage, is given in Table 3.10. It was not simply the issue of the separation from the family, but the effect on family life, the change from term times to holiday, and the effect on siblings. This is discussed in more detail in Chapter 8. For none of the parents we spoke to would boarding have been

Table 3.10. *The numbers attending a
boarding school for the deaf at each stage*

	Number	%
Infant	13	16
Junior	17	21
Secondary[a]	33	40

Note: [a] This includes one who became a boarder
during her secondary school career.

an expected part of their lives, if they had not had a deaf child. Boarding
just did not fit in.

*Schools are not available for them to go to, so if you like it or not,
they've got to go away. You've no choice in it. I did say to Miss ..., in all
fairness, that there are children who are simply not residential material.
There are parents that are not residential parents and we are two of
them. We didn't want him to go.*
Mother of Terry, 22 years, oral

She could not tell us what was happening but she was not happy

We did not include any specific questions on teasing or bullying. In
retrospect we wish we had, as it was mentioned spontaneously in a number
of interviews.

*He did like it but he was bullied. He had some bullying from the hearing
pupils. He has some unhappy times.*
Mother of Colin, 24 years, BSL

*Father: We had one or two problems at school, when he was at school,
where they began to take the mickey out of him, and he got injured then.
Interviewer: Did he? Actually physically injured?
Father: Physically injured...Stitches.*
Father of Phillip, 19 years, SSE

*She was bullied at S... School. She used to come home with black eyes
and bruises. She could not tell us what was happening but she was not
happy.*
Mother of Marion, 19 years, BSL

*He's not told us, it comes up months later. He has come home with his
hearing aid damaged. He would always come home with a bleeding ear
if he had had any impact on his head. You can't protect him 24 hours a*

day. The only thing you can stop is if there is bullying in a group. I think there is a danger you can be over-protective for the wrong reasons.
Father of John, 22 years, oral

We have no way of knowing whether these are isolated incidents, whether deaf children are more or less likely to be teased or bullied than hearing children or the type of settings that lead to the most bullying. Nevertheless, regardless of the extent of bullying, its consequence in terms of suffering in the incidents reported cannot be ignored. Because it was not fully addressed in the interviews, we did raise it in one of the group discussions. Of the five in the group, two could recall incidents of teasing or bullying at school involving both themselves and other deaf pupils.

I was young, I'd be playing outside in the playground and the hearing children would come up and wave their hands around and go on about deaf people being stupid. When I went to the secondary school there were a lot of hearing children; we felt the deaf children could not get back at them and we got teased every day.
Paula, from group discussion

There was a person that would always tease me. He would wave his hands around and my friend and I used to get very.very frustrated, very cross, but we had to be patient, and then the next day this person would do it again. And in the end I got really mad and I ended up putting my hand through a glass door with frustration and I ended up in hospital.
Phillip, from group discussion

For one of the young people an incident that could have been interpreted as teasing seen by her as a form of support.

I was at school, the first year at comprehensive school. I had a radio aid and I used to test it with the teacher's mike. I would leave it on her desk. My hearing friends would go up and sort of test it going, 'Testing, testing, one, two, three' before the teacher arrived. When the teacher came they would sit down quickly. So my experience is that they were aware of deafness, and I'm pleased, because they sort of supported me, in a way.
Carol, from group discussion

The other two in the group did not feel they had been teased or bullied.

They expected too little of me
Young person

Table 3.11. *Parents' satisfaction with education by stage of schooling.*
This question was answered by 81 parents of children at infant and
junior stages and 82 at secondary stage

| | Infant | | Junior | | Secondary | |
	Number	%	Number	%	Number	%
Satisfied	50	62	52	64	40	49
Dissatisfied	16	20	13	16	19	23
Mixed feelings	15	19	16	20	23	28

They didn't seem to stretch them enough
Parent

The parents in describing their satisfaction with the education that their
sons and daughters had received, talked of each stage of schooling
separately. A summary is given in Table 3.11.

Parents' responses also tended to suggest that more of their children
were unhappy at secondary level than at primary level. Almost twice as
many young people were described as 'unhappy' or having 'mixed feelings'
about secondary school as were so described at primary level. This is in
keeping with the tendency for parents themselves to be less satisfied with
secondary education than they had been with primary.

This was in contrast to the young people's reports. When they were
asked at what stage of schooling they were happiest, ten of them replied
that they were always happy at school and one that they had never been
happy at school. Of the other 48 who were able to answer the question,
seven were happiest at the infant stage, 13 at the junior stage, and 19 at the
secondary stage. For the other eight, it varied within stages. Thus the
secondary stage was the most popular with those specifying a stage of
schooling. We feel the difference between parents and young people relates
to the different factors operating. A number of parents described that while
their children were young they had seemed like other children; as they
became older differences became apparent and it was necessary to consider
the implications of deafness for the future.

Interviewer: Was there a time when you were feeling particularly
unhappy?
Mother: Towards the end of his education.
Father: Yes, well, that was the implications then.
Interviewer: So that was when it hit you...?
Father: Yes. I mean you realise the implications then because you have

got to think, right, if he's going for a job, who's going to go with him, who's going to read the papers for him?
Mother and father of Phillip, 19 years, SSE

The young people, however, seemed to find it more difficult to cope at the early stages of schooling but had adjusted by the later stages and were making friends and developing relationships.

While overall most parents and young people were generally satisfied with the schools attended, a common complaint by both groups was that not enough was expected of the young people, academically, at school.

In talking of their son's academic experience in a special school this mother noted:

I do think that teachers for the deaf, once they are qualified, they are too complacent. I felt this in the E... school and in the D... school. I used to go into the E... school and they would always be doing the same thing, and talking about the same thing. They didn't seem to stretch them enough.
Mother of Gary, 20 years, oral

And this mother notes, of a Partially Hearing Unit:

He (the Head of the Unit) kindly looked down on them. He did not expect much. He was upset if they could do more, because they had no expectations of them.
Mother of Helen, 23 years, SSE

And of a mainstream placement, these parents commented:

Father: I think we were so relieved that she seemed to be fitting into a reasonably normal hearing environment that we perhaps didn't really pay much attention to detail about her progress that we might have done.
Mother: No I don't think we...we didn't take enough interest in what she was learning. How she was getting on. There again when we asked, it was, 'Oh she is all right', and that was all we ever got. 'She is all right; she is happy'. That kind of attitude that this child is handicapped (and) if they can keep her reasonably contented they are not bothered about anything else. And in fact this is an attitude we have come across with an awful lot of parents who have not bothered to try and push the child to do more. Their attitude has been, hasn't it, 'Oh this poor thing, he is deaf, lets keep him happy and as long as he is, don't worry. Can't be bothered to try different kinds of education – haven't done anything.
Parents of Carol, 23 years, oral

A most damning indictment occurred when a parent was discussing her son, who was at college, studying drama, and a very successful student. His ambition was to teach and he would be qualified to teach drama. She asked the head of service, in the authority in which he had grown up, if he would employ the young man when he qualified.

> *So I said, 'Would you be prepared to employ him on your team, if you like as a peripatetic teacher?' and he said 'No'. He wouldn't do it. () And he is the boss of M... Hearing Education (service for hearing-impaired children). So that was interesting! Because to my way of thinking: I won't accept the fact that Phillip, because he is deaf, has got to go and work in a factory or a mundane job, which is what happens to the majority of deaf people we know. But that is the expectation.*
> Father of Phillip, 19 years, SSE

The young people themselves commented on this 'under-expectation' at school.

> *It was boring at W... school. The teacher wrote on the board and we just had to copy it. It would be all right if the teacher would talk first and then we wrote, but it was boring copying the board all the time.*
> Harry, 20 years, BSL

> *They expected too little of me. I think so. I don't think any of them expected too much. I think I had to prove them wrong...it is the image. Deaf child – she hasn't got any ears – she can't hear – she won't be able to do a lot of things, you know. A lot of people weren't sure. But all the way through I have proved them wrong. You just have to be determined.*
> Ruth, 19 years, oral

> *Staying there for five years (referring to secondary school) was a waste of time. The teachers were not bothered, they wasted my time. They were not bothered about history or anything. They wrote on the blackboard and then sat and read the paper.*
> Paula, 24 years, BSL

The young people were asked whether too much or too little had been expected of them at school. It proved a difficult question to answer, and only 31 of the group gave a response. Of those replying, 12 thought the expectations were about right, 11 that they were too low, and seven that they were too high. One said it was different at the different schools attended.

There were some young people who were satisfied.

> *It was all good. At first I wasn't sure it was the right school (referring to secondary school) but now I am older I'm pleased I went there. There were more people, lots of different subjects. It was very strict but that didn't bother me. It was close, like a family.*
> Isabel, 21 years, SSE

And some that felt the education they had had was too demanding.

> *They expected too much, perfect behaviour. We had to do everything right.*
> Deborah, 20 years, oral

The young people who felt too much was expected of them were usually referring to schools where there was an emphasis on oral skills.

I am not satisfied with his reading and writing

Reading and writing were often matters of special concern and many parents felt they were not taken seriously enough.

> *I will tell you why I wasn't keen on that school. He could read but he didn't understand what he was reading! When I pointed this out to them, they looked at me and said that of course he could. Well, anybody can learn to read, but he didn't know what the words meant. When I used to say, 'Well, what is that?' I mean he had no idea! He knew how to read but he wasn't gaining anything, because what he was reading was just words. They had taught him to read, but he didn't understand it. And that panicked me in a way. I thought, 'This is no good'.*
> Mother of Mark, 20 years, oral

> *I am not satisfied with his reading and writing. My son (11 years old) is better than him.*
> Father of Anil, 23 years, BSL

For these parents their son's first report issued when he was 16 years old was a real shock.

> *This was his first report. And his reading age at that time was 9.8, and his vocabulary age was 7. () His written language – it says, 'Phillip's written language is poor'.*
> Father of Phillip, 19 years, SSE

Later in the interview his father commented further on these low expectations.

*That's the level they expect, you see. ( ) Well, they have said to me that he
has reached above average say for a deaf person. But to me that's not
good enough. We shouldn't say, 'Well, its good because it's average
with the deaf'. We should try and improve it so other good lads can rise
to the top.*
Father of Phillip, 19 years, SSE

On leaving school, as with many in the sample, Phillip's reading ability was
not good, and he was not able to read a newspaper without help.

Parents were asked about their sons' and daughters' attainments and in
particular about their basic literacy skills. The majority of the young
people were described by their parents as competent (26, 32%) or adequate
(37, 45%) at reading, 'competent' meaning the young person could read
well with understanding, and 'adequate' meaning their reading ability was
generally sufficient for their day-to-day lives. However, 14 (17%) were
described as poor readers usually reading only single words or headlines
and five (6%) were completely unable to read at all. Thus only one-third
were competent readers and one-quarter were functionally illiterate.

The parents were also asked about their sons' and daughters' ability to
write. Only 18 (22%) could write with ease, meaning they could write a
letter to a friend with no help, although a further 34 (41%) could do so with
help. Nearly one-third required a great deal of assistance in writing (25,
30%) while 5 (6%) could write nothing at all. Thus the findings for writing
were more depressing than those for reading.

Parents were also asked about basic numeracy. One-third of the young
people (29, 35%) were considered competent, a further 44 (54%) having
adequate skills for day-to-day life. Of those weak in this area, 7 (8%) were
described as having poor numeracy skills and 2 (2%) as having no skills at
all.

These results are consistent with research studies that have tested the
literacy and mathematical skills of deaf school leavers. Conrad (1979), in a
classic study, demonstrated a median reading age of nine years, and it
appears from inspection of his data that 40% were functionally illiterate –
a more pessimistic figure than that suggested by this research which may
indicate an overall change over time, or may reflect either differences in the
way of assessment, or differences in the sample examined. Conrad only
considered those leaving specialist provision for deaf pupils, although a
greater proportion were in specialist provision then than now.

The mathematical competence seemed to be the most positive result
obtained in this research, with only 10% being not competent at all and
over one-third being competent. This greater competence is also indicated

Table 3.12. *Achievements in public examinations by the young people.*
(The parents were reporting on the period prior to the introduction of
GCSEs.)

	CSE	GCE	A-level
None taken	28	68	75
Sat, none passed	10	2	1
1–2	14	3	5
3–4	15	1	1
5+	15	8	0

in the work of Wood, Wood & Howarth (1983) who found mathematics
ages of 12–13 years in deaf pupils in their final year at school.

As well as in reading, writing and mathematics we looked at the formal
attainments of the group in public examinations. The achievements of the
young people in the study are shown in Table 3.12.

Overall, of those who achieved success in public examinations, either
CSE, GCE or A-level or a combination, two-thirds had success in subjects
which included academic subjects, while one-third had success in only
practical subjects. Because of the age range of our group of young people,
comparisons are complex, but as some indication: of the general population in 1988/89, 22% of males and 23% of females left school with one or
more A-levels, compared with 7% of this sample. In 1985/86, 13% of males
and 10% of females left school with no externally examined qualification,
and in 1988/89, this dropped to 10% of males and 7% of females (Central
Statistical Office 1992). This compares with the 46% of our sample leaving
school with no such qualifications.

Of the sample, eight eventually went into higher education, one to
university, two to polytechnics and four to colleges of higher education. Of
these, one used BSL, two SSE and five were oral.

BEYOND SCHOOL

I was uncertain about the future

I was happy to leave

Because school systems differ from county to county it became apparent
that to ascertain the age at which the young people left school would be
extremely complex. It was decided that if a school had an integral sixth

Table 3.13. *Age of young people on leaving school*

Age (years)	Number	%
16	57	70
17	10	12
18	9	11
19	2	2
20 or older (stayed on in special unit)	4	5

form or a sixth form college, offering for the most part O- and A-level opportunities, then the young person attending such a school was considered to be still 'at school'. If the young person entered a college or further education department, integral to or separate from their school, offering among other things a wide range of vocational courses, then he or she was considered to have left school and entered 'further education or training'. Training is considered further in the next chapter. These criteria must be borne in mind when viewing Table 3.13, which shows the age of leaving school. It can be seen that the young people in our study did not tend to stay in conventional schools beyond the age of compulsory schooling; 70% were considered to have left school at the age of 16 with only 11 (14%) staying on to the age of 18 years.

Interestingly, while the parents often spoke most vividly of their feelings about their son or daughter starting school, the strong emotions for the young people were focused on leaving school. For them, it seemed to be leaving school that, at the time we spoke to them, evoked the most vivid memories, both of happiness and unhappiness. It may have been the structure of the interview or the importance of recency for the deaf young people. For those leaving schools for the deaf, in particular, it could mean leaving a world of deaf people for the hearing world. Overall, slightly more were pleased to leave (21, 46%) than were negative (16, 35%). The others had mixed feelings (9, 20%). For 15 the question was not answered.

I wanted to go back to school. All my friends were there and I wanted to stay there for ever.
Darren, 22 years, SSE

I was worried, uncertain about the future.
Amanda, 20 years, SSE

I was upset, I cried, I missed all my friends.
Richard, 20 years, oral

However, there were just as many who were happy to leave.

I was happy to leave. I felt more relaxed in home and work surroundings.
Tom, 20 years, BSL

Relief. I went home happy. I did not enjoy school.
Shirley, 22 years, SSE

I felt glad to leave school, and join the hearing world. I was very nervous, though, that my contact with the deaf had finished.
Christopher, 21 years, BSL

CHAPTER FOUR

The world of work

There is no progression in the job. Ideally I would have liked her to have had a job which she could have really enjoyed, where she could have progressed and earned a decent salary. It took a long time before we realised we were just dreaming. It just wasn't going to be reality. You start with such high hopes for your children. It took a long time to come down and accept that was all she was going to do.
Father of Fiona, 22 years, SSE

The period when the interviews were carried out, coming as it did when the young people were between 18 and 24, with most in the 20 to 22 age range, came at a time of transition, in terms of both working and social lives. This chapter is about the choices that were made around leaving school, entering work and/or training and deciding about future careers. Table 4.1 shows the status of the young people at the time of the interviews with both the parents and with the young people. These figures form the basis for much of the information in this chapter, therefore both sets are presented.

On first inspection, this would seem to paint an optimistic picture. Two-thirds of the sample were in employment and less than one in ten were unemployed. Figures such as these, showing as they do a picture of apparently high levels of employment, conceal a less encouraging picture of frustration and disappointment. Many parents felt their sons or daughters to be underemployed and not to have jobs that matched their capabilities. Many of the young people felt themselves to have had little opportunity to determine their own career path and to be in the wrong job. Families often felt that the advice they had been offered was poor, and the preparation of the young deaf people for life beyond school, inadequate.

The quote that begins this chapter was chosen, not because it was

Table 4.1. *The circumstances of the young people at the time of interview*

	Parent interview		Young person interview	
	Number	%	Number	%
Employed	53	65	43	70
Full-time education	7	9	7	11
Unemployed	7	9	5	8
Job scheme	6	7	3	5
Sheltered workshop	4	5	1	2
Life skills course	3	4	1	2
Rehabilitation unit	1	1	0	0
Caring for child	1	1	1	2
TOTAL	82		61	

exceptional, but because the concerns it contains were expressed in a variety of ways by many of the families in our interviews. The account of Isabel's life, which introduced the whole book, also described a young person whose abilities were not fully utilised. The hopes expressed are not out of the ordinary or over-ambitious, in fact they are the sort of hopes that any parent might have for a son's or daughter's working life. Yet all too often these aspirations seem not to have been realised.

THE BEGINNING OF A WORKING LIFE

As an introduction to the issues, we describe the experiences of Wayne. While the combination of events is unique, no one particular event is unusual. It is by no means the most depressing story; many worse things happened to others in the study. However, the account does give some indication of the effort that can go into finding work, the unfair treatment that can be meted out, and the frustration and distress that this can cause.

At the time of the interviews Wayne was 21 years old, and he communicated orally. He had both deaf and hearing friends, though most of his life was spent in the company of hearing people. He got on well with his parents and brother, often went for a drink with his friends and to discos at the weekend. He passed some CSEs, but in practical subjects only. He passed his driving test first time when he was 18 years old. Before he left school, he had had work experience in a brewery and a farm.

While at school, he had attended an interview at the local Careers Office, where they had asked him what he liked doing. On the basis of this, it was suggested that he considered working in a bank, an idea which his parents found entirely inappropriate. He was keen to leave school and his first position was in a YTS (Youth Training Scheme) painting and decorating scheme, from which he received good reports. Right until the last day he was told it would lead to a permanent job. Two days after he should have finished, his mother rang the YTS office to find out what was happening. They rang the firm to find that it could not afford to keep him on, but the boss would be telling him that day.

> *So of course he comes home for his lunch break whistling and singing. I thought, 'He seems happy today' so I let him sit down and have his meal. 'Have you seen the boss?' 'No, not yet, () he will be back at tea time to tell me what is happening.' I said, 'I am sorry, Wayne, but I am afraid you are finishing tonight'. Tears he had then. Then he gets angry, tears and then angry.*

There was then a period when Wayne was receiving Social Security payments. He then applied for a painting job, which he had seen advertised. After some delay, during which he was interviewed twice, he started work, but it only lasted two days.

> *Wayne had got his back to him (the boss) and he said something Wayne did not hear, so he shouted and said, 'Are you bloody deaf or something?' () Then he shouted bad language right down his hearing aid. Wayne said, 'Really bad language', he couldn't repeat it. So he did no more, he told the other lad he was packing it in. () The chap said, 'Oh, if you can't take a bit of bad language' and Wayne said, 'Well, there's language and language'.*

Then he went on a Young Workers scheme where the pay was low, the Government paid half and the employer half, making it less expensive for the employer. He was again painting and decorating which he enjoyed, though working 12 hours a day for minimal wages. By the end of the six months, he was totally responsible for painting an Indian restaurant on his own. Then one day, he came home late.

> *He said, 'I was just finishing off the job there or nearly finished it and he (the boss) comes to me and says, 'I want a word with you'. I thought he was going to give me my overtime but he says, 'After next week I don't want you any more, because your work's no good.' () So he (Wayne) told the Indian bloke, 'You won't see me any more after next week'. He said, 'Why not?' Wayne said, 'Because the boss has finished me'. He said, 'What for?' Wayne said, 'He says my work is no good'. He said the man went up the wall. 'My word your work is first class. You come to me for a reference.'*

After this Wayne went back to receiving Social Security payments again. He disliked the Social Security Office. He was reluctant to go there on his own as he had to write everything down and the officials did not have any patience with him. Usually his father accompanied him, a situation which his father recognised was degrading for Wayne. At this time his parents actively encouraged him to look for work.

I said, 'Look, Wayne, it's up to you, you have got to start writing letters. Look, let's write a list of firms' and I wrote a list of firms for him. () And I would go off to work and say, 'I want to see some letters on there when I come back'. And he had done them, nice and neat () but I came in one day and he was just watching television, you know, messing about. I said, 'You have got to do something, write some letters'. 'I am fed up with writing letters.' I said, 'If you are fed up with writing letters get on your bike and go round the firms'. () 'I will tomorrow.' I said, 'All right, tomorrow then, whatever the weather get on your bike and go'. I remember saying it to him. And it chucked it down with rain and I made him go. () But you know it was heart breaking, because he came back.

At every place he had gone to he had been told that he had to write a letter first – so it was back to writing letters. The parents were very worried about his long-term prospects.

I had visions he was not going to get a job. And Greg used to say, 'Why will they employ him when he is deaf, when they have got all these others?'

After a time, because his mother was concerned about him, she rang the Careers Office again.

He was upset he was on the dole and I rang up the Careers Office and said, 'Look, I know Wayne is really over the age now', I said, 'really he has been let down on two schemes', can he help? He said, 'Let him come down and see me'. He had an interview, came back and he said, 'I don't know what he was on about – he was on about some scheme'. I says, 'My word, he better not be!' He says, 'I couldn't understand it – he is going to ring you anyway'. He did ring me and he said, 'I don't know whether Wayne has explained to you what I was trying to tell him, but there is a scheme where they all do the sort of things they like, painting, electrical work. () I said, 'Look I am very sorry but Wayne has been on two schemes already; it is time he had a job – and better paid.' He said, 'Well, it would be good for him'. I says, 'Look, no way is that lad to go on a scheme again!'

There were a couple of jobs the family heard about but they were not suitable for Wayne; one was at a foundry and the employers felt there was a safety risk, the other involved the use of the telephone. His parents were upset at the way this particular situation was handled, because Wayne had made it clear on his application form that he was deaf. They telephoned to invite him for interview but when his mother explained he could not speak on the telephone, they just said to tell him not to bother to come for interview as he needed to use the telephone for the job.

Then he went to an interview for a labouring job. He took all his references along, and they asked why he had come for that when he was too well qualified. He explained it was all he could get. They said they could offer him something better and put him in the stores, where he was working at the time of the interview. There was evidence he was teased at work, although it did not appear to have been an issue for him.

> He came home from work the other day and one of his mates had stuck a leaflet on him that should have been stuck on the wall for some reason. To me I thought, 'They are taking the mickey out of him' but he didn't mind that, he thought it was funny.

The parents were asked if he was happy at work.

> I don't think so. He does now and again come out with funny things like – more money – or another job, but we just let it slide.

He had been there for three years at the time of the interview, and his employers seemed to be pleased with him. The employer has said to the parents.

> 'I wish I had got more like your lad,' he says, 'He does keep working. Others are playing about but he keeps working all the time'.

However, there was a threat that the workplace might be closed. The parents dreaded him being out of work and having to start the search again. They felt that on the whole, Wayne had not realised his potential, yet they did not undervalue his successes at work. In describing the way he had coped at a course he had had to attend, they said:

> We are very pleased. Sometimes I think we do not give him enough credit for what he has done. I don't think we do. People come and tell me, 'I think he's great'. Then sometimes I feel quite chuffed with him.

The issues raised by this account are among those discussed in the rest of the chapter. The lack of careers guidance or appropriate guidance and difficulties in obtaining work are illustrated. It shows how training schemes, rather than providing training and access to work, could be a barrier at which deaf young people could become stuck, receiving little or no training yet working a full day for minimal pay. Even when work was obtained the jobs could be unsatisfying and the lack of recognition of potential, frustrating. It is also clear from this account that parents may come to take a significant role in assisting the transition into work.

VOCATIONAL GUIDANCE AND CAREERS ADVICE

You just don't aim high. That was bred into us without our knowing.

Guidance about careers can be informal in terms of general discussions and work experience, or formal involving interviews with Careers Officers or school staff who have that specific responsibility.

Many of the young people (44/58, 76%, three did not answer) had had work experience which, for the most part, they valued. Most of them advocated it as good policy for deaf pupils who are about to leave school.

> *I went to... Building Society for one day a week for a year. It helped me build my confidence and get used to mixing with hearing people.*
> *Isabel, 21 years, SSE*

Even a less positive experience can be beneficial.

> *I spent two days a week at... Hotel, in the laundry. I did it to get away from school. I learnt that hearing people talk about deaf people behind their backs – and that I did not want to work in a laundry.*
> *Zoe, 19 years, BSL*

Another young man saw the benefit of work experience, not as being for himself, but because it educated hearing people about deafness.

> *Yes, because a lot of hearing people think that deaf people do not work hard. If there was more work experience they would realise that deaf people do work hard.*
> *Gary, 20 years, oral*

More formal guidance was less common, though. Of the 54 answering the question, only 16 (30%) could recall any formal guidance being given, although 25 (46%) reported discussions at school about work and work situations. Much of the guidance was, however, negative and focused on what the young people could not do rather than what they could.

I wanted to be a car engineer but Mr... said it would be too hard, because of my deafness; it would be better to do other engineering, such as street lamps.
Harry, 20 years, BSL

I wanted to work in the ironing press, but the man who helped with the deaf visited me at home and said ironing was not for me. Then he helped me find a job in a handbag factory.
Diana, 20 years, BSL

I wanted to be a teacher, but the careers officer asked me how I thought I would cope, how I would use the phone in emergencies. He made me feel really uncomfortable. () I gave up the idea of being a teacher during my A-levels.
Deborah, 20 years, BSL

First at school, we didn't have a very good careers service. It was appalling as a matter of fact. We had two careers teachers and they weren't dynamic enough, they didn't give us the information. () Second, they had very low expectations of deaf people. 'Oh, you should go into jobs where you don't have to use the telephone, where you are not responsible at all.' That's a fact. I can't describe it. You just don't aim high. That was bred into us without our knowing.
Janet, 22 years, oral

I would have liked more idea of what people in my situation could do. The careers teacher was not very helpful. At the careers interview they told me I would never get on a Nursery Nurse course and that I should train to be a chiropodist. I proved them wrong.
Louise, 22 years, oral

In fact not only did she get on a Nursery Nurse course but she got the highest marks in her year.

Many of the parents were concerned about the inadequacy of the careers advice and guidance. Almost a third (25, 30%) of the young people in our study, as far as their parents were aware, had not received formal guidance, either at school or afterwards. A further third, (26, 32%) had had some guidance at school only, 13 (16%) had had guidance after school only with 18 (22%) being advised both before and after leaving school. We asked the parents' opinions of the quality and usefulness of the guidance received by the young people, irrespective of the stage at which it had been given. Nearly half, 47% (27/57), of parents were dissatisfied with the extent and quality of vocational guidance received and a further half (28/

57, 49%) were only moderately satisfied. Only a small minority (2/57, 4%) were fully satisfied with the advice received.

> *He was no help! I mean he just kept saying, 'What do you want to do?'*
> *and Nigel said 'Book-keeping', and he said 'Right, make sure that is*
> *what you do do!'*
> Mother of Nigel, 19 years, oral

> *Of course, when he left school, he went for the careers interview at 16.*
> *'Your child won't work, you realise! There is no work.' That was the*
> *careers interview!*
> Mother of Darren, 22 years, BSL

As in the example cited at the beginning of the chapter, some careers advice seemed inappropriate. In other cases it seemed to parents that Careers Advisers had preconceived notions about the types of jobs deaf people could and could not do. The parents reiterated the young people's concerns about the negative quality of much of the advice.

> *They didn't give her any ideas to better herself – just destined to do*
> *menial tasks. She would have liked to have been a hairdresser – they said*
> *it was no good because she has to talk to people.*
> Father of Marion, 19 years, BSL

> *Most things that were suggested that Amy would like to do it was, 'No,*
> *no you can't do that', because of her hearing problem.*
> Mother of Amy, 19 years, BSL

> *She wanted to work with children. () We were told at these career*
> *conferences – 'No way!' She loves children. She is very good with*
> *children. Could she not work with handicapped children? 'No!' They*
> *were very defeatist, I suppose. We came away feeling very miserable.*
> *They kept on about factory work. I didn't want her to work in a factory.*
> *That seemed to be what they expected. It was traditional.*
> Father of Fiona, 22 years, SSE

> *Father: She applied to three colleges and was accepted at all three with*
> *the minimum requirements. An excellent achievement to actually go*
> *for three interviews at three different colleges and be accepted by all*
> *three.*
> Mother: Especially as the advice was that she shouldn't take up teaching
> *and that she perhaps wouldn't get into college.*
> ()

Mother: Ruth was upset because they had intimated to her that, well, did she really think that she could teach? And she was very upset.
Parents of Ruth, 19 years, oral

Ruth was successful in her application to train to be a teacher.

As well as poor-quality advice, lack of information was a serious problem for the young people, some of whom said they felt ill-informed, and had little idea what they wanted to do.

I did not try to get a job in engineering, but the school picked it for me. I was surprised. I did not know what I wanted to do.
Charles, 20 years, BSL

I didn't know what I wanted to do. My mother had to help. She picked typing. She said, 'I think you should learn typing'. I didn't really like it at first but it's all right now.
Helen, 23 years, SSE

The hearing pupils had a lot of information, but it was more difficult for me; there wasn't enough information. Most of the information I got was from my family.
Phillip, 19 years, SSE

As illustrated by the last quote, it was often the family who gave advice and support. Having little expert help to guide them, parents themselves had to take on the role of adviser, though some resisted giving advice:

I think let them find out on their own what they want to do, what they want to settle down to, rather than say to them a) you have got to do this or b) you can't do that because you are deaf...I wouldn't say to Sharon, 'You have got to do this when you leave school because there is nothing else you can do because you are deaf!' I think you have got to let them find their own way and what they want to do in the capacity that they are able to do.
Mother of Sharon, 21 years, BSL

Parents felt that the dearth of vocational guidance provided before and after leaving school often meant that their children had no ideas at all about what were feasible or possible occupational options. Over one-third of the young people were described by parents as having 'no idea at all' about what they would like to do after school or college. It seems clear that the young people were not well served by experts in terms of guiding them towards a career. Often limited work opportunities had their roots in the lack of careers advice, or the poor quality of advice, together with low

Table 4.2. *Highest level of education completed or in progress*

	Number	%
Full-time higher education	8	10
Full-time further education	24	29
Full-time further education, course not completed	2	2
Work-based training scheme	19	23
Day release	4	5
Apprenticeship	2	2
Correspondence course: professional qualifications	1	1
Life skills course	3	4
Rehabilitation Unit	1	1
No training	18	22

expectations that they had received. In some instances, it seemed that their sons and daughters had no ideas at all and the very people who could have been broadening horizons and suggesting possibilities were those with the lowest expectations of the deaf young people, yet because of their position were seen as knowing what was best.

> *These people do seem to get it in their heads what they feel would be best and expect everybody to go along with that.*
> Terry, 22 years, oral

The situation seems to have changed little since 1958, when the following was written:

> The need in some areas for better co-ordinated placement scheme, including vocational guidance is an urgent one. Boys and girls leaving school for the deaf have little idea of what their vocation is, or of the countless openings for the deaf in a complex industrial society, or of the different types of training scheme available, or of the general organisation of factories and other units.
>
> Drewery (1958), quoted by Rodda (1970, p. 38)

EDUCATION AND TRAINING

They didn't know how to communicate with her

Increasingly, as the demands of the work situation grow more complex, the need for training and post-school education becomes more important. Table 4.2 shows the level of education and training reached by the sample,

Table 4.3. *Type of college attended by the young people*

	Number	%
College for deaf people	6	11
Unit for deaf people at mainstream college	2	4
Unit for disabled students at mainstream college	7	12
Mainstream institution with other deaf students	13	23
Mainstream institution alone	25	44
Combination	4	7

based on information from the parents' interviews. The interviews revealed that 57 (70%) of the young people had had, or were still receiving, some form of college-based post-school education or training. Table 4.3 shows the type of college they attended. Where deaf students were accommodated in colleges for deaf students, but were going out into mainstream colleges for their courses, they were considered to be students of the latter rather than the former. It is interesting to note that the majority (38/57) of the young people entered mainstream colleges and for the most part (25/38) they were not placed with other deaf students. Of those attending a mainstream institution alone, six were at places with previous experience of deaf students and 19 where there was no previous experience.

Sometimes the lack of awareness of deaf students was disturbing.

> *The college was not very good, not very helpful. I couldn't understand the teachers – they left me alone and I couldn't get on with the students. One, I couldn't understand what he was saying, his mouth was very small and he did not help me.*
> *Amanda, 20 years, SSE*

And efforts to help could misfire.

> *She (a social worker) made all my lecturers come to a meeting one lunch time and they were sat at this big round table and I didn't want to go because, I mean, how would you feel with all those lecturers looking at you, if you know what I mean.*
> *Interviewer: So you were there?*
> *Yes. I didn't want to be there. It was a bit patronising but she made me go and I had to tell them what I felt and I had to say, 'You shouldn't do that and you shouldn't do that'. And I was only 20, I think I was, I was shy of doing it and all these lecturers all these intelligent people. I should have made the most of it but...*
> *Janet, 22 years, oral*

Both parents and young people appreciated a college situation where communication was easy. In one instance, it was described as the best part of the young man's education.

I think probably now (is the best time). It's college. Right now he can talk with his tutor. The tutor can sign and he can talk with him. He can have a proper conversation. He couldn't have a proper conversation with the teacher in the Partially Hearing Unit. There is no way he could have a proper conversation. I think because Phillip wasn't fluent (in English) and she couldn't sign. () Its a whole new ball game for him, really it is.
Father of Phillip, 19 years, SSE

Where there was not this support, parents were critical.

He was with hearing people, and they did not know what to do with him. He just sat in the corner and read a book all day.
Mother of Douglas, 22 years, oral

She had day release once, but the college did not know she was deaf. () They were all in a room talking and she did not have a clue. This woman tried to take her out in a room on her own but she couldn't explain, and that was no good. Somebody came to support her, that was once, but it was hopeless. They were talking about computers and banking, but she did not have a clue what they were talking about and what it had to do with her; overloading and loadsharing. They didn't know how to communicate with her.
Mother of Marion, 19 years, BSL

We were interested to explore how well the young people felt they were supported in their post-school education. A higher proportion (48/61, 79%) of the young people actually interviewed had experienced post-school education than in the total sample based on the parents interviewed (57/82, 70%). They were asked first whether they had an interpreter or communicator who attended classes with them to interpret or explain. Of the 44 who answered, 34 had experienced such support, 33 from teachers or communicators and one from a social worker. Of the other ten, nine said it had not been needed. While this appears to indicate high levels of support, when we asked about its adequacy a less optimistic picture emerged. Of the 30 who answered, six felt the support they had had to be completely inadequate in terms of the amount given and its quality. A further 14 said that the support itself was good but the amount received was inadequate and only ten were satisfied with the support. We also asked about other forms of support, notetakers, lip speakers, radio aids and

Table 4.4. *Support at college*

	Notetaker	Lip speaker	Radio aid	Extra tuition
Always or regular	5	6	2	13
Occasional	13	6	3	6
Never	19	28	36	19
Not answered	11	8	7	10

extra tuition and the results for this are given in Table 4.4. Of those with notetaker support, in ten instances it was a formal provision and in eight it was other students.

We asked the young people in general terms how friendly they had found the other students (hearing). Of the 42 who answered, 16 (38%) felt they had good relationships with other students, 22 (52%) mixed, and four (8%) found other students not at all friendly.

Other students? Not very well. They frightened me. They wouldn't talk to me.
Amanda, 20 years, SSE

There are 17 in my group. Four are OK with me, two are really helpful, one asked me out for a drink once.
Keith, 19 years, BSL

Interviewer: Did you go out with the others?
No. No I didn't. I just used to go to college and come straight home.
Josie, 24 years, BSL

Because in our pilot interviews, some young people had indicated to us that they were not adequately prepared when they went to college, we asked specifically about this. Of the 31 answering this question, just over half (17, 55%), felt they were ready and 14 (45%) felt they were not ready, mostly (11) because of a lack of necessary skills in English.

I wasn't ready for the course. I couldn't answer some of the questions – I could not understand all of the words. English is at the root of all the problems.
Christine, 21 years, SSE

In looking at post-school qualifications obtained, because colleges offered such a vast array of internally and externally examined courses and parents' own knowledge was sometimes vague as to the exact nature of the examination taken by their son or daughter, it was decided to simply record whether the young person had passed college-examined or

Table 4.5. *Who had helped young person in search for a job*

	Number	%
Self only	7	10
Family or friends	35	50
Parents	26	
Other relations	5	
Friends	4	
Professional	27	39
Disablement Resettlement Officer	19	
Further education staff	8	
Other	1	1

externally examined courses, or a combination of such courses. From parents' responses it seemed that of the 57 young people who had attended some form of post-school education, six had attended college without any consequent examination success, 13 had received only college-endorsed certificates, 17 had passed externally endorsed courses only and ten had passed both internally and externally endorsed examinations. Eleven were attending college but had yet to take examinations. Almost one-fifth of parents commented spontaneously, when interviewed, that whilst their children had passed practical examination papers with ease they had failed or had to retake theoretical papers.

FINDING EMPLOYMENT

Every job I've got or ever had, has been through my Mum or Dad

For the 70 (85%) young people who were in, or had been in, some form of employment, job scheme or sheltered work we asked who had played the greatest part in finding and obtaining that position. Table 4.5 based on the parent interviews shows who had helped in this. Six of the seven unemployed are included here, as two had previously worked, and four had previously been on job schemes. In addition, the young woman caring for a child had been on a job scheme.

Thus, while for 39% of the young people, a Disablement Resettlement Officer or further education officer was felt to have been responsible for finding their current placement, for half the young people, the family and friends were important in this. The example at the beginning of this chapter illustrated the major role parents could play, as do the following examples.

I think it was her Dad and I that really () I mean, I sat down with her one afternoon when she was on holiday and said, 'I think we should write some letters now to the banks and what have you' and I said to her, 'Write to the Post Office', and she said, 'I have written to the Post Office once,' and I said, 'Come on, let's write again!' So she did it again.
Mother of Isabel, 21 years, SSE

Yes, I took it on my own back. I took him to the S... firm, you know, just before he got his community scheme a year ago, because he fancied working in the soap works and doing nights – he wanted to do a night shift for some reason, you know.
Mother of Tom, 20 years, BSL

I got an advert for this job from the local paper; we looked night after night, Helen and myself. We wrote off to British Airways, Castle Donnington Airport. We wrote to the Gas Board, the Electricity Board, the Railway – you name it, we wrote! Must have written 40 letters, always with a CV – she did that herself, typed it out, all her certificates, all the work she had done, and those were sent off with a letter.
Mother of Helen, 23 years, SSE

We went to the job centre and didn't get any help at all. Dave was working for the District Council and he knew of some places available. He actually brought some papers home. It was clerical. It was YTS. She got an interview and I went with her as an interpreter. She got the job.
Mother of Amanda, 20 years, SSE

One mother reported her daughter's dissatisfied feelings on the matter:

She said, 'Every job I've got, or ever had, has been through my Mum or Dad!'
Mother of Louise, 22 years, oral

Sometimes we think it's degrading for him, having his Dad there

Parents often felt that their children needed an advocate at interviews or at the very least some form of communication support. We asked if such support had been provided and who had provided it. Table 4.6 summarises the support at interviews described by the parents for the 62 who had had interviews and for whom this information is available. As can be seen from this table, once again parents were most frequently named as the providers of communication support.

Table 4.6. *Support at interviews*

	Number	%
Parent	34	55
None	20	32
Social worker	6	10
Friend	1	2
Interpreter	1	2

I think some employers think, 'Oh, if she is deaf she might be daft'. The ones at P... because when I went for an interview with her, she couldn't understand the lady that was interviewing so I had to go and help. ( ) She got on fine then.
Mother of Mary, 23 years, BSL

When she got the interview I went with her and made sure they knew she was deaf. Nicky was fairly recalcitrant at the job interview. She was very lacking in confidence, they sensed that, and they asked me if Nicky was lacking in confidence or is it because of the job interview situation? I said that she is a confident person in herself and she doesn't think she'll get this job because she is deaf! She got the job!
Mother of Nicky, 21 years, SSE

Not all parents were happy with this level of involvement, feeling it to be intrusive and humiliating for their children.

Another (job) we went for was a garment factory where he would have to stick labels on. But he never got...He was interviewed, I went with him and answered the questions by interpreting between us. There has always had to be a third party there. ( ) I suppose there always has to be a third party to be able to understand what is going on. Although at the same time I think Phillip would cope. They would have difficulty if they couldn't sign and they couldn't talk. ( ) Sometimes we feel it's degrading on Phillip's part, having his Dad there.
Father of Phillip, 19 years, SSE

Although the ideal situation may seem to be to use a professional person to interpret, this was rarely experienced, and not always seen as successful. One young person felt that the presence of an interpreter hampered their job chances.

My first interview I failed, because I had a social worker as an interpreter. I think it makes hearing people feel I can't communicate

without an interpreter. I went on my own this time and got the job.
Christine, 21 years, SSE

I've had five years of these schemes and I've had enough

The Youth Training Scheme started in 1983 as a one-year programme, and developed into a two-year programme in 1986, just before the interviews for this study took place. It was intended as a programme for young people offering them vocational guidance and training. Although it was an improvement on the previous Youth Opportunity Programme, which came to be seen as using young people as cheap labour, it never became the major programme it was originally intended to be, and many young people remained sceptical as to its value. It has since been superseded. Also operating at the time of the interviews were a variety of other schemes, including the Community Project Scheme, which involved youth, who might otherwise not have worked, in community projects.

Of those who had left full-time education, over half (46/75) the young people had experienced YTS or Community Project Schemes, with a small number (six) still remaining in such situations. This was greater than the proportion for young people as a whole. The National Youth Cohort Study, at around the same time, showed one in three young people spending time on such schemes (Courtenay, 1989). Given that such schemes were created to enhance entry into the real job market, it was disturbing to discover that over half (25/46) had experienced two or more schemes, with three having experienced four or more schemes.

One criticism of them was that they gave little training and were often seen as exploitation.

> *He is on a community programme for one year. He has done 11 months, so he only has one month to go. He's achieved nothing on it. He's not got any kind of training whatsoever. He's doing joinery. They make toys.*
> *Mother of Matthew, 21 years, LLS*

Parents became very impatient with offers of such schemes.

> *He's been on the Community Programme for a year, and then on the dole, and then on the Community Programme for a year, and then on the dole!*
> *Mother of Darren, 22 years, BSL*

> *Cleaning the churchyard, it's ridiculous, it's not for him, but because he's hard of hearing he's put in the Community Task Force...Commu-*

nity work for three months and then they gave him another. Three times he was on the task force.
Mother of Douglas, 22 years, oral

I have had enough of these schemes. I've had five years of these schemes and I have had enough.
Mother of Matthew, 21 years, LLS

For some, however, the YTS placement led on to employment.

He went on a YTS course straight after school. He was there for about three months and then he got a chance to go to a firm called H... and B... He was one of the YTS lads. The manager was told that Sam was profoundly deaf and he was willing to give him a chance for a week. When that week passed he gave him a trial for 12 months. Once three months had passed he was making the window frames and he signed him on.
Mother of Sam, 18 years, BSL

Of the six young people in schemes at the time of the interviews it was felt that four would be offered more permanent positions in the companies within which they were placed.

UNEMPLOYMENT

No chapter on work would be complete without some mention of the unemployed, those young people who were unable to find work. As mentioned at the beginning of this chapter very few (7, 9%) of the young people in our study were formally unemployed, two women and five men. Of these seven, five had never been in employment at the time of the parents' interviews, although one had found work by the time she herself was interviewed. Of these five, three were young men and two were young women and they ranged in age from 19 to 22 years. One was a BSL user, one SSE, two were oral and one had limited language skills. Four had previously been on job schemes. Direct comparisons with other studies of youth unemployment are difficult, because of the age range in this study and the varying ways in which data are collected in the different studies. However, approximate comparisons can be made. The overall unemployment rate in 1989 was 7.1%. However, for young people, the rate was higher: for males, 16–19 years, it was 12%, whereas for older males, 20–29 years, and females 16–29 years, it was 9% (Central Statistical Office, 1992). A comparison can also be made with the National Cohort Study, which at

Table 4.7. *Unemployment*

	Number	%
Never	33	40
Insignificant	13	16
1 period	17	21
2 periods	9	11
3 or more periods	3	4
Full-time education	7	9

a similar time found 9% of young people to be out of work (Courtenay, 1989). Such data suggest that the rate of unemployment of the young deaf people was consistent with national trends at the time.

The unemployment experience of the group is shown in Table 4.7. Our concern here is to demonstrate not only those who had experienced unemployment but also those who had a number of periods of unemployment interspersed with periods of work. A period of work or unemployment is taken here to be of at least two months. The category 'insignificant unemployment' means that for less than 5% of the period since leaving school the young person was out of work.

Over half of the young people had never been unemployed for anything other than insignificant periods. However, over a third had experienced periods of unemployment, and 4% three or more such periods. The National Cohort Study found that 14% had experienced periods of unemployment, although the data are not directly comparable, as the period here was six months. While it is not possible to say whether this is a comparable figure, it does seem that a large number (29) of young deaf people had experienced significant unemployment.

THE EXPERIENCE OF WORK

The first day at work must have been terrifying

For many of the young people transition into work was a dramatic one. We asked the parents who had done the most to prepare the young people.

Oh us, me and her Dad. Oh and her older sister helped tremendously. We feel she brought Sharon out of her shell in many ways. Sharon used to be very shy and she has always been able to go to her elder sister and talk things over, you know, how sisters talk. Actually she has been fantastic with her.
Mother of Sharon, 21 years, BSL

I think it must have been quite a shock to Isabel when she started work, because up to then she had had quite a lot of people helping her and sheltering her, particularly when she was at secondary school. She was very much protected, I would think, and then all right when she left there and went to college it wasn't as sheltered, she had to be more independent then. But then finally I think it hit her when she came home and she got a job and she went out there. They had never employed a deaf person before and she was on her own. I wasn't there, her Dad wasn't there, she was there on her own. That first day at work must have been terrifying.
Mother of Isabel, 21 years, SSE

I'd like to stay here, climb the career ladder, build on what I've done

It's a very boring repetitive job

For the most part, at a superficial level, it seemed that most of the young people who were working were happy at work. Two-thirds (29/43, 67%) described themselves as happy at work, 5 (12%) were happy but had some problems, and 9 (21%) were unhappy. The ones who were the most satisfied were those who felt their abilities had been recognised, often by promotion.

I am very happy in this job. I got promoted last week to quality inspector. In the next three weeks we have 1000 printed circuits to set out, though. To some extent I can now please myself what I do. I'd like to stay here, climb up the career ladder, build on what I have done.
Malcolm, 22 years, oral

On the first day I was nervous but after that it was OK. () I would like to stay here for ever. They've asked me to become a supervisor. It might be difficult if a lot of people come in. I am the number one worker, though. Most people can only work one machine but I can work them all.
Richard, 20 years, oral

Having someone who could communicate easily with them was also a major positive factor.

When I started work I was surprised to find there was one man who could sign, as he had worked with a deaf person before. He helped with any communication problems.
Andrew, 21 years, BSL

However, further probing and more detailed questions revealed a more complex picture. Although they may have been happy at work, 23% (10/ 43) complained of low pay.

> *I make wooden boxes to send round the world. The money is no good. I would have liked to go in the army but I couldn't, because of my deafness.*
> Douglas, 22 years, oral

> *I like the job but the wages are low. () I looked first for a job with good money, but I couldn't find it so I came here.*
> Charles, 20 years, BSL

Some of the young people felt they were being paid less because of their deafness or that they were generally exploited.

> *In the job before, I found out that the boss was paying the others more than me. I did not find out until later, because I was deaf. I went to see the boss and then he agreed to pay me more.*
> Dennis, 19 years, BSL

> *I get blamed all the time for any bad work. They think I am thick, because I am deaf, but another lad works with me and some of the bad work is his. They pick on me, make me sweep up, it's poor wages.*
> Harry, 20 years, BSL

Dissatisfaction also arose from the fact that they felt themselves to be in a job they disliked.

> *I have a job printing balloons. It is a very boring repetitive job.*
> Rachel, 22 years, BSL

> *I work in a shop, a bakery, but I don't like it. It's washing up all the time and being a general help, not bakery. I have to get up at five every morning, which is tiring.*
> Ann, 21 years, BSL

One young woman had wanted to go into computers but had been made to feel she would not be able to do this. Instead she was encouraged to train as a hairdresser, but as she points out hairdressing has many disadvantages for deaf people.

> *It was pretty difficult for me, it was hard.*
> *Interviewer: What was hard?*
> *Trying to communicate. Washing – talking to the back of their heads because I couldn't really hear what they were saying. They were talking*

in the mirror and I was washing their hair and I couldn't really – I didn't – it was difficult – I didn't really feel comfortable. That's why I finished in the end.
Josie, 24 years, BSL

A further major cause of dissatisfaction was boredom with the work and a feeling that they could do more. The young people were not expressly asked about whether or not they were understretched in their work or job scheme, but nine (9/46, 20%) spontaneously mentioned it. Our data suggest that slightly more than half of those in full-time employment or job schemes (30/59, 51%) were understretched, according to parents.

He was under the understanding when he went there that he was going to do a little food preparation – kitchen assistant type of thing, but instead of which they gave him the job as the washer-upper and he had to do a split-shift system. () All he was doing was washing up and never had a break and he used to go seven days a week. () At the end of it he just got absolutely sick and fed up with it. My husband went down to see the manager there and asked him if there was any chance of a proper job and he said, 'Well it is a new venture, none of us really knows. It depends how it takes off'.
Mother of Christopher, 21 years, BSL

She has just recently applied to change; to sort of move upwards, if you like. () She is now bored with what she is doing, because it isn't demanding enough.
Mother of Paula, BSL, 24

However, by the time of the interview with Paula herself, the promotion had been achieved, but only after her own strenuous efforts.

I have promotion. I went to the interview and I said I wanted a transfer to somewhere else. The boss was very surprised that I wanted to leave so he offered me a better job in a different department. I couldn't believe it. I had had a big argument with him last year.
Paula, 24 years, BSL

The people at work make me frightened

With the benefit of hindsight, we regret we did not explore teasing and bullying in some detail. The only question we asked related to this concerned the extent to which the young people felt talked about behind their back. We made it clear we did not simply mean that conversations went on that they could not hear, but they felt the fact they were deaf was used by others to allow them to discuss them in their presence. To the general question, 'Do you ever feel people are talking about you?', 23 of the 46 in jobs or job schemes (50%) specifically mentioned work as a situation in which they felt talked about.

There were more serious examples of teasing and bullying, though, and although there were no questions specifically using these terms, it was mentioned spontaneously by a number of both parents and young people as a source of concern.

I used to get teased. The boys there cut my shirt. They were stupid. I was cross and told the boss, and two of them were suspended in three days.
Gary, 20 years, oral

I was teased in the factory, so I left. I work in the foundry now and they leave me alone...They used to call me deafy and stupid. They didn't bother with me. I wanted to teach them to sign, but they don't want to. I sit by myself at break times, eat sandwiches and drink all on my own. I'm bored. I'll stay here, because my mother and father want me to. I'll stay until I'm 65.
Ivan, 21 years, BSL

When people swear at me and call me names I want to walk out, but my Dad says I have to stay here. Today at work the others told me to get lost, they are horrible to me. The people at work make me frightened.
Douglas, 22 years, oral

Sometimes the parents were aware of this. In the account that introduces this chapter, the parents commented on the label being stuck to their son's back. Other examples could be more extreme.

He has a lot of bullying. () The fact he was deaf and therefore he was an imbecile.
Father of Daniel, 21 years, oral

They call him 'shit face', terrible. I keep saying to him, 'They do that anyway' but there is no need for it, in my opinion. It doesn't seem to get any better.
Mother of Andrew, 21 years, BSL

He got a lot of bullying. Once he got roped up by the legs, over a beam, and hung up by his leg. Once he got a dart right in the back of his head. It was because he couldn't stick up for himself.
Mother of Matthew, 21 years, LLS

At P... he was being ragged, this boy disliked him and it came to blows. This boy was a trouble maker. Nick wasn't the first boy he'd had a go at, it came to blows so they sacked them both instantly. He was being teased about his hearing aids but the worst thing was he got hit over the head. He did the appeal bit but it didn't work. ( ) They got the union on it but if they gave Nick his job back they'd have to give the other his job back. He'd been there two years. He'd worked all the hours God sent, he'd never got into trouble for being late, he'd worked Saturday, Sundays.
Mother of Nicholas, 24 years, oral

She was actually trained for more than she is doing

Whilst these young people for the most part entered a saturated job market where almost every job advertised attracted an abundance of qualified and over-qualified applicants, it seemed to many parents that the odds were set against their offspring, even when they had endorsed recognised qualifications. Parents described their daughters and sons as having a sense of missed opportunity; a sense that had they not been deaf more interesting and more challenging options might have been open to them, as the description of Isabel's life, which opens this book, suggests.

One of the young people in our study had gained a national prize for work she had done as part of her college B.Tec course but found herself, in what she hoped would be a temporary position, vacuum-packing kitchen doors in a factory. Her father remarked regretfully,

Having done that (college course) she can't get a job. She's got a Higher B.Tec. in Production Design but she can't use the phone so can't take instructions verbally, so she's going to be difficult to employ.
Father of Brenda, 21 years, SSE

Another gained a Nursery Nursing qualification, after being advised she would not get on the course (see page 96). After qualifying, she found herself offered a classroom assistant post, which she found unstimulating. She could have taken up such a post without her hard-earned qualifications.

She was disappointed that the jobs she was going for were not real jobs. Having come out of college with this qualification she couldn't get the job she wanted.
Mother of Louise, 22 years, oral

Both Brenda and Louise had found jobs by the time they themselves were

interviewed, although after considerable effort. By the time of the interview with Louise, she herself had got a better job, although it was not the
job she really wanted.

*I tried lots of jobs, I knew it could be difficult. I wanted a small firm as I
knew it would be easier for communication. I have a job now, though I
really wanted product design. () My father's friend advised me to work
there for the summer, then they offered me the job...I like it but I don't
want to stay there for ever.*
Brenda, 21 years, SSE

*I always knew I wanted to work with children, but it took me three
years to get a proper nursery nurse job. I stopped putting I was deaf in
the application form – just let them find out at the interview. I have only
just got the job I want, though.*
Louise, 22 years, oral

DEAFNESS AND WORK

If she hadn't been deaf the sky would have been the limit

In an account such as this, it is difficult to specify the extent to which it is
deafness that has affected the working lives of these young people. While
deafness as an issue pervades most of the accounts, some of the experiences
of these young people and their families would be shared by hearing young
people starting work at the same time. Poor careers advice, difficulty in
obtaining work, training schemes that do not lead to permanent jobs and
poor career prospects are not unique to deaf people. The statistics on
unemployment and training schemes are not out of the ordinary.

Yet most of the young people and their parents were in no doubt that
their working lives had been affected by the deafness, in almost every
respect. This chapter has described a group of young people, most of
whom are in work, but when we look at the finer detail in the picture,
rather than the people in it being satisfied, many of them are variously
bored, frustrated, angry, and disappointed. Few of the young deaf people
in our study received the quality and extent of vocational guidance they
required to allow them to develop informed choices about career options.
Where they had no ideas of their own, they were dependent on their
parents' interest, knowledge and experience, and the advice of their
teachers and careers guidance officers. Many potential employers showed
ignorance and sometimes discrimination; looking for the most part at why

they could not, rather than how they might, employ the young deaf people; the emphasis was on what they thought the young people could not do, rather than exploring what they could do.

It should be remembered that these young people and their parents were not living lives in isolation from the community at large, they knew about work and employment possibilities. In most families (76/82, 93%) there were hearing siblings with whom comparisons could be made. Parents felt that deafness could influence opportunities at the application stage and the interview stage and perhaps most of all it appeared to affect the type of job the young people could expect.

> *Interviewer: Do you think he would have been in this job if he had not been deaf?*
> *No, he wouldn't have been. He wouldn't do it now if he could get out. He takes after my husband. I think he would have got to university because things click so quickly with him.*
> *Mother of Andrew, 21 years, BSL*

> *If he had his normal hearing, what he wanted to do: he wanted to be a courier with several languages, you see, travelling around. () He loves driving, you know. I mean he can drive and what have you. He passed his driving test in London, so that is no mean...He would have loved to...something simple like driving round on a coach or something all over the world with his little mike there.*
> *Mother of Mark, 20 years, oral*

> *I think if she hadn't been deaf, the sky would have been the limit, because she is very bright. She would probably be doing something outdoors but she would have done something entirely different. She has mentioned the army. She's not stretched enough. She needs more stimulation, more mountains to climb.*
> *Mother of Nicky, 21 years, SSE*

As the quote above indicates, there was one particular exclusion which was a disappointment to some of the young people – the Armed Services.

> *I am always trying to prove myself. If I was hearing I would have gone into the forces, marines or paras, but I don't talk about it now because it depresses me.*
> *Jeremy, 20 years, oral*

> *I had always thought of joining the Navy but I went for the interview and it got as far as the medical, but I couldn't do it because they thought I was too deaf to join up.*
> *Michael, 20 years, oral*

Even so, one might feel that sometimes unrealistic aspirations play a part, that deafness is taking the blame for something that was inevitable. It could be said that many young people desire to do things that are outside their capabilities and that many have to compromise their aspirations, taking less than desirable jobs. Modelling and acting are cases in point.

I want to be a model. I have lots of books about modelling. I have a book of photos of me, modelling. I was the only deaf person in my group to do this. I would like to work in the future but I am not sure I will get it, because I am deaf.
Shirley, 22 years, SSE

There is however, evidence that deafness affected the type of work attained. Although social class classification can only at best provide an approximate measure, it can give some indication of the status of work obtained by the group. Of the 59 young people in our study who were in work or job schemes, one was classified as Social Class I or II, 12 as Social Class IIIWC, 23 as Social Class IIIM, 16 as Social Class IV, and seven as Social Class V (Registrar General Classification). Most of the young people in our study held manual and unskilled positions. In fact, over half of the young people were in one of six broad types of work: clerical or office (8, 14%), manufacturing industry (11, 19%), car mechanics (4, 7%), joinery (2, 3%), warehouse work (4, 7%), or catering (2, 3%).

We felt there was, in fact, evidence of underemployment and under-achievement in the sample. We took a crude measure by comparing the work status or educational attainments of the young people with those of their siblings (where there were siblings and they were of appropriate age). For these 65, it seemed that 12 (19%) of the young deaf people in our study occupied a position with equivalent status to their siblings, 36 (55%) occupied a position with a lower status, 4 (6%) of the young people were in positions of a higher status, with the remaining 13 (20%) having some siblings occupying positions of lower and some of higher status. Therefore over half of the young people were in positions of an inferior status to that of their sibling or siblings.

As soon as they knew he was deaf they didn't want to know

The restrictions in the choice of work available to the young people is compounded by the fact that few employers have experience of deaf people and know what to expect. While some are positive and open, many are negative and some afraid. Excluding those in sheltered placements (eight) or still in full-time education (seven), the parents of one in seven of the young people (10/67, 15%) felt the attitude of employers was a major and significant barrier to obtaining work or work progression. In many instances this seemed to be because of fear or ignorance.

This woman at the R... Centre went with Rachel to the interview and Rachel came back and told me that the man who was interviewing them was frightened of her. You know he said, 'I have never had a deaf person come before' and she reckoned that spoilt her chances. She said he looked frightened. He didn't really want to talk to her.
Mother of Rachel, 22 years, BSL

None of the firms'd touch him. () He'd go to an interview and as soon as they knew he was deaf they didn't want to know. Personnel departments ought to be educated or someone ought to go with them... nothing like this at all.
Mother of Douglas, 22 years, oral

He did go for an interview with the social worker to C... and he was very disappointed, because that was the sort of job he wanted and everything was fine. () But the boss couldn't understand what he said and he wasn't prepared to...I mean you can do after a few weeks, you can understand what Robert means. But they hadn't got the time.
Mother of Robert, 22 years, BSL

Some places just took one look at him and didn't want to know him. This was most places. We went for other jobs before. He applied to pubs, hotels, odd-job work. The sort of work he went for was totally labouring and the reaction he got from most places was disgusting. They didn't want to know once they knew there was something wrong with him. And that's the hotel industry and pubs who pay very low wages, employ people to peel potatoes in kitchens at night, even those sort of people didn't want to know him.
Father of Alistair, 21 years, oral

I took him for this interview and the personnel manager was saying there is no detriment really because he is deaf, but there is a hazard. I think they were a bit scared really, because I thought probably he could have found him something.
Mother of Tom, 20 years, BSL

Somebody as bright as Phillip and he could not fill a shelf

Alongside fear and ignorance were the perceived consequences and the stereotyped expectations of deafness. These arose both from employers and from professionals in the field of deafness. Some of these have already been discussed in terms of the advice given. One mother was even told at the time her child's deafness was diagnosed, of the expectations she might have for him.

> *We took N... there and had him tested, and we were told he was profoundly deaf, 'But don't worry, he can grow up to be a cook or a carpenter'. That really upset us. I can remember the tears streaming down my face. It was awful, it was demoralising.*
> *Unattributed*

This young person has recently graduated from University.

Excluding those in college or sheltered placements, the perceived consequences of the deafness were felt by nearly two-thirds, (42/67, 63%) of parents to have influenced job chances. Perhaps the most frustrating effect of deafness on the work process was that once the young people were in a job situation the families felt that they had considerable difficulties in making progress or gaining promotion. Of the 40 (13 had been in work for less than a year) who had been in permanent work for over one year, even if they had changed jobs during that year, only eight (20%) had progressed to a higher status position, while 32 (80%) remained at the same level of work.

> *Interviewer: What is preventing him move up? (...)*
> *I think it would be his deafness. Perhaps they don't feel he is capable. I said to Harry, 'Do they know you have been on a computer course?' and although it (the computer course) wasn't very long at all they say he took to it like a duck to water, you know. He was really quite good on it. I think they are just apprehensive – they feel he is not capable. But I said we can't as parents, we can't go to the firm and say, 'Give him a chance'; he has got to do that himself.*
> *Mother of Harry, 20 years, BSL*

> *There's no chance of job prospects. It's obvious people are going to select a hearing person as opposed to all the difficulties a deaf person has.*
> *Mother of Hugh, 20 years, BSL*

The most commonly mentioned specific barrier to progress was the telephone. An inability to use the telephone prevented the young people from applying for many jobs and also from being promoted within jobs. This was a factor in the account described at the beginning of this chapter, where Wayne was told on one occasion not to bother going for the interview if he could not use the telephone. Other young people had similar experiences.

It is purely her deafness that will hold her back, because there are certain things she can't do. It is an impossibility. She can't use the telephone. () She could never go onto a job where the phone needs to be used quite regularly and at (...) these are the most important jobs. () She could never deal with the public. This is where they earn most money, you see. That is what Isabel is interested in. () You see where she is now at (...) they are very reluctant to give her different jobs, because they are wondering all the time, 'Can she cope with it?' and 'How are we going to cope with it if she can't?' This is it – it is communication.
Mother of Isabel, 21 years, SSE

There are lots of jobs she can't do, because of not being able to use the telephone. Actually when she had to leave C... they did get her interviews with two or three other departments and they did say that had she been able to use the 'phone one of the jobs she could have had.
Mother of Carol, 23 years, oral

Until recently the telephone was the only way of communicating quickly and at a distance, but now with the growing use of interactive computer communication networks and fax machines, as well as text telephones developed especially for use by deaf people, perhaps it will not be long before the telephone as a barrier to employment will not be so pervasive.

Problems in communication were also mentioned as making some employment impossible. While this may be the case for some types of work, in other instances the excuse seemed a little far-fetched.

Before he went to college, when he left school, there was an advert in the paper. () He went along and he had an interview at A... and it was filling shelves. () (She said) she couldn't employ Phillip because he would have to talk to the customers. Sometimes the customers would ask one of the lads or girls, 'Where are the baked beans? or say, 'This orange is mouldy!' or something like that. So she couldn't employ him to fill shelves. Well, I was devastated. Somebody who was as bright as Phillip couldn't fill a shelf!
Mother of Phillip, 19 years, SSE

Employers often cited the potential dangers in the workplace as a reason for not employing deaf people. Not being able to hear the fire alarm was one of the most common examples given, although while some firms saw this as insurmountable, others found ways around this difficulty. Other potentially dangerous situations were also cited.

I got a full-time job as laundry assistant, sorting out clothes. I wanted a job with the machines, putting clothes on hangers. The manager said I was not suitable, because I was hard of hearing. He would talk to me and I could not hear him so he said it was not a suitable job, because of safety.
Daniel, 21 years, oral

I had a bad experience at one interview. They said they did not want deaf people in the workplace. I asked why deaf people could not do engineering, deaf people can see, its just they can't hear.
Keith, 19 years, oral

Another reason given was the danger not only to the person themselves but to others. The following young woman, having gained a Nursery Nursing qualification, after initial difficulty in convincing vocational advisers she should train, had the following experience at a job interview:

She did apply for a job on the wards – that wasn't a very good experience either, because they knew she was partially deaf. At the interview the lady that was interviewing her put her hand in front of her mouth purposefully. Why I don't know. So Louise couldn't catch anything she was saying. It was on purpose to see whether Louise could actually hear the children. Louise said she wasn't a very sympathetic person. On the other hand when she went up to a ward for a day, to see how she could cope, the sister said she would have loved her, because she was very good. But because of the risk there might be to a child, if Louise didn't see them, because you have to have, as you well know, you have to have eyes in the back of your head almost to keep up with them. If Louise was not facing the child and something happened to them then there was a risk there. But she said that Louise was more than capable of doing the job.
Mother of Louise, 22 years, oral

It would be difficult to deny that there is some employment which is unsuitable for deaf people, in the same way that most people could specify work for which they themselves would not be suited. Our concern is that often the reasons given seemed to be a consequence of lack of information and of stereotyped expectations rather than based on a clear appreciation of the situation. While there may be barriers to the employment of deaf people in some situations, our feeling is that these are far more limited than some comments would indicate.

In carrying out the interviews we were struck by the contradictions in career advice and work practice, in that barriers that seemed insuperable to some were ignored by others. One young person was advised against hairdressing (page 97) while another was actively advised to take it up despite her lack of inclination (page 111) and she did find it unsatisfactory. One young person was discouraged from teaching and gave up her ambition while another successfully applied for and completed a teacher training course. It is disappointing that often low expectations were endorsed by the very professionals who were expected to assist deaf young people.

Well, there's nothing to be worried about, because I can cope with that anyway

We would like to conclude with two examples of work choices that may be seen to be unsuitable for deaf people: a swimming-pool attendant and a stone mason. Yet in both these situations the young men involved have been successful.

At the interview I said, 'I'm partially deaf and I'm not bothered about it, but if you're bothered then I'm walking out', and they asked me to stay. I explained what I could and could not do. They arranged to help me with special alarms and so on. I am very vigilant at the poolside, I watch all the time. () I like doing the out-of-pool attendant duties, working in the bar, switching off the lights, picking up the rubbish, but I can't do it at the same time while I am doing poolside duties. I have to watch all the time.
Unattributed

Well, I heard about the job when I was at...College; it was a magazine that comes out every month.
Interviewer: All about stone masonry, was it?
It was a stone industry magazine, designed particularly for the outside industry, and I applied for it and I got a letter two weeks later saying would I come for an interview () and he said, 'I don't think there is anything wrong with your attitude to work, it's just we are a bit worried about your deafness'. () Well, the most important thing he worried about was safety, because the fact is you have to be able to hear shouts or anything falling, so that you can stop yourself from getting hurt. () I said, 'Well there is nothing to worry about there, because I can cope with that anyway'. () It is very interesting and also you are saying you are putting something back into a church or something and you will say, 'That will be there for another 200 years before it is replaced!' It is going to last longer than you are and you know your children or my children will say, 'Look' or 'My Grandad did that'. It is quite fascinating.
Unattributed

CHAPTER FIVE

Deaf young people in a hearing world

Later on in life, you get more and more things you don't know what to do and then I ask my father what to do and then I know what happens in the future. Its like when there's an accident or something like that happens in the house – I don't know how to claim insurance. Or I have to ask my mother and she'll explain about the mortgage level, or phone and they'll send me a form to fill in and it's clear and I fill it in, but first I show mother and see if it's right because it's the first time I've filled one in.
Paula, 24 years, BSL

From their teens onwards, young people in general are increasingly expected to take control of their own lives and manage their own affairs. As well as being a time during which they are starting training or work and developing their social lives and relationships (both dealt with in other parts of this book), they are becoming increasingly independent in the areas of shopping, housing, banking, travel, medical care. Young people usually get support in this from their families and their peer group as well as information from the media and from schools and colleges.

Developing independence requires increasing interaction with institutions and organisations within the hearing world. However, this world is by and large ill-equipped to respond to deaf young people. Few hearing people are aware of the implications of deafness and BSL is still not recognised as an official language in this country, although it is recognised by the European Parliament. With few exceptions, little is done to ensure that the information and services deaf people need are accessible to them.

This chapter continues the theme of the last chapter, the transition into adult life, by looking at areas of autonomy in the public domain and about how this is achieved. In this context it considers the aids and equipment that are available to deaf young people to facilitate communication and access to information.

SHOPPING, BANKING AND INSURANCE

I didn't realise what it meant and my mother explained

One of the least problematic areas of all for deaf people is shopping, not because of the awareness of shop assistants, but because self-service stores minimise the amount of face-to-face communication required.

> *When she went to shop it would always be a supermarket or shop where she could take it off the shelf, go to the till, and she can look at the till, see how much it is.*
> Mother of Sharon, 21 years, BSL

The parents' accounts showed that while just over half the young people always shopped alone (51%, 42/82), over a third (31, 38%) would need accompanying for complex purposes, and nine (11%) never shopped alone. For usually competent deaf young people, it was sorting out hire purchase or similarly complex financial arrangements that were likely to require parental support or explanation.

> *We went to buy a fridge/freezer and it was very very difficult for him, because he was going to buy it on the weekly and I had to go with him to fill the forms in and it was rejected. ( ) But he couldn't grasp that. He said to me when we came back 'What about the forms for paying?' I said, 'You don't have to pay monthly, you have bought it, you have paid for it all now.' And he couldn't believe it. ( ) 'I don't know, I don't know how I have done that'.*
> Mother of Robert, 22 years, BSL

> *When they moved into this flat they had to fill in a form to say they'd only just moved in and the rates did not need paying until...and that sort of thing, and they got a bit worried about that. Also they had an estimated electricity bill because they hadn't been there, and they were both a bit worried that it was more than it should have been so I showed them how to read the meter and send the card back and then they would send another bill with it done properly.*
> Mother of Josie, 24 years, BSL

And one mother told how difficult it was to explain to her daughter, who, having experienced buying one thing interest-free, wanted the same facility for her washing machine.

> *She asked, 'When can I go in and have the six months' free interest?' and I said, 'Well, you can't go in and say you want it, it has to be on offer' she said, 'What do you mean?' I said, 'Well, like in the paper, if you see "ON OFFER – 6 MONTHS' FREE CREDIT" you can go in, but you have to pay it in the six months'. She didn't understand at first. I had to keep going over it. She sort of realised.*
> Mother of Rachel, 22 years, BSL

Many parents pointed out how the language of the hard sell, 'free offer' 'win a prize, no strings' could be especially confusing for deaf people, designed as it is to be misleading to the hearing population.

> *The 'Club books' that's the worst. When it comes through the door and it says, 'This colour set's yours, free'. The first word they look at is 'free' and the next one is 'colour television set' 'name and address'. They fill it in and send it away.*
> Mother of Shirley, 22 years, SSE

> *Well, there are two planes. He knows more about money management than I will ever know but he really has not reached the responsible stage. We have had on more than one occasion to bale him out when he has run up hundred pound bills with the Readers Union and things like that. He is very vulnerable, it seems. He is easily swayed by glossy adverts.*
> Mother of Francis, 19 years, oral

The intricacies of banking services are not always easily mastered by the average user and certainly for the young people in our study parents often had to explain certain banking procedures or become involved in advising on managing finances. Whilst 87% (71/82) of the young people had their own bank accounts, only 43% (35/82) of the young people managed their finances completely alone; the remaining 57% (47/82) needed some degree of parental help.

> *My husband is trying to educate him now. He is trying to do everything by direct debit, standing orders for his mortgage, and everything. We try to persuade him to put money in the building society and do it all himself, but he is finding that a hassle. He doesn't want any hassle, he says, for the first year he is going to do it all by standing order and direct debit, you know. So he is having to cope with all of that, but we have just had a hiccup on that, which he would have sorted out for himself but there wasn't enough time, so I had to go and sort it out for him.*
> Mother of Colin, 24 years, BSL

Table 5.1. *The relationship between preferred language and the ability to manage own finances, and the ownership of bank accounts*

	BSL	SSE	Oral	LLS
Manages own finances	12	6	17	0
Does not manage	19	7	13	8
Own bank account	29	12	28	2
No bank account	2	1	2	6

With his bank book he has got at L... he couldn't understand it, how every so often he got his...and he pointed it out, interest. 'I never put it there'. You sort of have to take a lot of time in explaining to Christopher that there is interest on that amount of money. Then he wants to know what interest is and what it is for and that sort of thing.
Mother of Christopher, 21 years, BSL

The preferred language of the deaf young people was not a major factor in either owning a bank account or managing their own finances, as shown in Table 5.1, except that none of those with limited language skills managed their own finances and only two of the eight in this group had their own bank account.

In managing finances, the issue was not totally or even predominantly one of being able to communicate directly with banks or other institutions, but one of access to information and understanding the concepts. The following excerpt from one of the group discussions illustrates this further.

Phillip: Talking about insurance, when I first bought my car, my father went to look with me; the second time my father said, 'Try it'. I tried it with the man – no problems. If it had been a different man I'd have had problems, but the same man explained the forms, because he knew I was deaf, it was the second time, it was all right because we had a relationship. If it's the same it's all right; when it changes to new people then I can't do it, it's a problem.
Carol: I had to insure our house contents recently, the price was too high. I asked my father to check the old one, there was something wrong, so my father phoned up for me and asked about the long words that are difficult. Sometimes I need help from my father and then I know what to do in the future.
Group Leader: That way you learn from father explaining different things so next time you know how to do it yourself.
Carol: Yes.
Group Leader: A lot of time in the school, maybe they didn't show you how to do things for yourself.

Paula: Not all of it, only part of it. Later on in life, you get more and more things you don't know what to do. Then I ask my father what to do and then I know what happens in the future. Its like when there's an accident or something like that happens in the house, I don't know how to claim insurance. Or I have to ask my mother and she'll explain about the mortgage level, or phone and they'll send me a form to fill in and it's clear and I fill it in, but first I show mother and see if it's right, because it's the first time I've filled one in.

Phillip: Or the first time you buy a new car and there's a problem like a question of salesmen speaking too fast and I can't follow him; it's like insurance or a mortgage, they see how much we are going to pay every month. If you buy a television or a car or things like that, sometimes its too much, then I'll ask my father for advice and he'll help me. I bought a video, the price was interest-free for ten months but the insurance you had to pay, I didn't realise what it meant and my mother explained. It's the same but she'll explain.

Interviewer: You said with hearing people you write, so why don't you go on your own for insurance and write it down?

Hugh: It's best to go with father, because my father understands more and with the forms the communication is very difficult. If you go for insurance the language is very difficult.

For all young people, learning about insurance, hire purchase and banking is difficult. Deaf young people, too, need to find out how the system works and what facilities are available for them. However, for many of them acquiring this information was not straightforward. It is easy to underestimate how much information is generally available to hearing people from a variety of informal sources. Many of the deaf young people did not have as easy access to information available in society through conversation with friends and family, through television and radio, or publicity material and advertising. We have already seen how being part of a group conversation could be more difficult for deaf people, and later in this chapter we discuss access to the media. Deaf young people may be less likely to read magazines or publicity material, and the language of finance is specialised, so it may be more difficult to access through the written word if the concepts have not been absorbed informally. Moreover, because most hearing people lack the skills necessary to communicate with deaf young people, and interpreters are not generally available, deaf young people were less able to consult advice services provided by banks, mortgage companies and so on. Most schools seemed not to have provided education in this area. All of this meant that the young people were often far more dependent on their families and in particular their parents for this information, on the very issues that are related to developing independence.

MEDICAL CARE

This is the place where you'd think people would know

Whereas banking, insurance and other financial matters are in the public domain, and taking a parent or friend along to assist may not seem too much of a problem, although it may represent an intrusion into private finances, going to the doctor's or dentist's is a more personal matter. From our mid-teens, we usually expect details of our consultations with doctors or dentists to be a private matter, which we may or may not choose to share with our families or friends. For young people, visits to the doctor may concern sexual or other intimate issues they prefer not to discuss in their parent's presence. Very few hearing people would want parental involvement in such medical consultations, but many of the deaf young people found that it was necessary for their parents or other family members or friends to accompany them. The parents reported that while over one-third (30/79, 38%) of the young deaf people in our study were able to consult their doctor alone, 34 (43%) required assistance for certain matters and 15 (19%) needed assistance at every consultation. Information was not available for three of the young people.

For some there was no problem:

> *I talk and if they don't understand I write it down.*
> *Paula, 24 years, BSL*

> *The doctor, I talk to him.*
> *Janet, 22 years, oral*

But for others this was not possible.

> *I don't understand the doctor. He talks too quickly and writes too-long words that I don't know. My Dad takes half a day off to go with me to the doctor's.*
> *Harry, 20 years, BSL*

> *There's sometimes a problem. I talk to him but it's hard to understand him. I take my mother or father. If it's private I go with father. It slows it down, having to write it all down.*
> *Darren, 22 years, BSL*

Sometimes the parent went because they felt their son or daughter would not be understood in a situation where understanding is essential.

I go with him to the dentist, mainly because he can't hear his name given over the mike. () He is actually due to go to the F... because he has some filling which keeps coming out; it is not drained off properly. I said, 'I will come with you, because I don't think he (the dentist) will understand properly'.
Mother of Robert, 22 years, BSL

Often the request did not come from the young people but from the doctor or dentist who felt that they could not manage.

In the past the doctor has phoned and asked my mother to come with me, so we can talk more. The doctor is frightened to talk to me on my own.
Isabel, 21 years, SSE

It's like Shirley being on the pill. () My doctor says, 'Will you always come with her, please? Don't send her on her own, because I shan't know how to deal with her. I've never dealt with deaf like this'. So I go and he asks and we do it between the three of us.
Mother of Shirley, 22 years, SSE

For parents of course this is a dilemma. Often they do not want to interfere in their son's or daughter's private life.

I take her to the doctor. You see, I should be saying, 'You go in, Isabel, by yourself, and try to make him understand what is wrong with you and see how you go. If you need me, then get someone to call me in'. But I haven't got the guts at the moment to do this with her. So what do I do, I toddle in with her, you see, and then what happens is, as soon as I am there he talks to me, you see, and I keep looking at Isabel, hoping that he will turn and he will talk to Isabel but no, he doesn't, he just continues to talk to me.
Interviewer: How does she feel about that?
She doesn't feel very nice about it, but I don't know whether this is my fault – maybe I should say to her, 'Go in and see how you get on. If you need me call me'.
Mother of Isabel, 21 years, SSE

He ignores Phillip and he only talks to me, but I think it's my fault again, because I should let Phillip go into the surgery by himself; then it would

be a one-to-one relationship and he would have to make himself understood.
Father of Phillip, 19 years, SSE

Many parents had consciously tried to assert their sons' and daughters' independence in medical situations, as emerged in one of the group discussions.

Phillip: Sometimes I might go to the doctor's and I used to take Mum or Dad with me and as I got older my Dad said to me, 'No you must go on your own; try by yourself'. My Dad wanted me to realise that when I got older I can't always take my Dad with me and he said he'd help me to learn to get used to going by myself and using pen and paper, so that was quite good really.
()
Hugh: Whenever I go to the dentist my Mum came with me and talked to the dentist, but now I go by myself.
Group Leader: Did your Mum tell you to go by yourself or did you say, 'I'm going to try'?
Hugh: My Mum said it was time for me to go by myself.

The dilemma for parents, of whether to get involved or not, is obvious when we consider these parents' comments about experiences on admission to hospital:

She went (into hospital) last year – kidney stones problems. One Saturday she was doubled up and she was sickly. Then the pain started. I went with her. She was very distressed that they couldn't understand her. They don't even listen when you go with her. I told the doctor when he came to see Amy that she was deaf. As much as you want people to use direct conversation to Amy, in this particular instance he was directing it to her and expecting an answer from her. It was far too technical. They couldn't understand her at all. I think it must be horrendous in these situations.
Mother of Amy, 19 years, BSL

And another example, this time where a parent wanted to explain her son's particular needs to medical staff:

He was lying there either asleep or with his eyes shut and I had to keep saying, 'Please touch him before you speak and then he will open his eyes' () they were saying, 'He won't come round', but they weren't touching him or anything. He wasn't coming round, because there was nobody getting through to him until I went and said, 'Look, he is deaf,

*you have got to touch him'. That is one place you would think people
would know. I mean it had got on his notes that he was deaf, because I
made them put it on.*
Mother of Nigel, 19 years, oral

We asked parents if they would feel it necessary to accompany their son or
daughter if they went into hospital to help with communication and two-
thirds (55, 67%) said they would do so. Many parents felt that they would
need to be with their son or daughter to explain to them the medical
procedures taking place.

The need to assist communication in medical situations may seem
strange, as there is a general expectation that medical personnel will have
some understanding of deafness and be able to deal with it. Often the
parents were accompanying the young people, not because they felt that
communication would be too difficult, but because they felt the professionals involved were not well enough informed or not prepared to take
the trouble to communicate.

COMMUNICATION WITH PUBLIC OFFICIALS

If the police stop me, I write it down on a piece of paper

Most of the young people in the sample had contact with various public
officials, including transport personnel, the Department of Health and
Social Security (DHSS), the police and social services. Nearly half the
young people managed this situation always or almost always alone,
although one in six (10/61, 16%) usually needed help. The other 26 (43%)
needed assistance with communication some of the time. We explored
further the need for communication support with the DHSS and the police.

With the DHSS, there appeared to be a procedure, although it was not
always clear.

If you don't understand you ask for form B1 and write it down.
Keith, 19 years, BSL

*Well, I couldn't manage it there (DHSS offices), because they had lots of
windows, and you had to shout through, and I couldn't hear what was
being said. I had to go up and say to them, 'Sorry, but I am deaf'. () In the
end it was easier to send the book to my home.*
Janet, 22 years, oral

My mother comes and the DHSS person talks to her.
Fiona, 22 years, SSE

A number of the young people had been involved with the police at some
time or the other. We are not here concerned with involvement in crime, as
the numbers of young people was so small as to be negligible. The issue
considered here is how the police interacted with young deaf people
whether they were actually charged, under suspicion of an offence or being
questioned as witnesses. Of the ten who had had some police involvement,
five were BSL users, one an SSE user, four were oral and none came from
the group with limited language skills. In only one instance did the young
people report to us that a professional interpreter had been involved. If
assistance with communication was required, it was almost always
provided by a parent.

If the police stop me, I write down on a piece of paper for them; they
phone my father.
Andrew, 21 years, BSL

When I was 16, I was on a motor bike. It had a broken light. The police
stopped me; I told them I was deaf and asked him to take his helmet off
(presumably for communication). Later my father explained to the
police and so they fixed my light for me.
Dennis, 19 years, BSL

The police caught me on top of a bus shelter; they were in plain clothes. I
pretended I did not understand.
Keith, 19 years, BSL

I lip read and then I write it down. I tell the police to come here (home)
with me and get help. They swear, they kick sometimes.
Darren, 22 years, BSL

I was arrested once. I was walking down the road, just walking about by
myself outside someone's house. They phoned the police. The police
came. I got them to phone my mother.
Miles, 20 years, BSL

They came about stone throwing. Mum helped me answer the
questions.
Edward, 23 years, oral

I interpreted for another deaf girl I saw in the street having problems
with the police.
Deborah, 20 years, oral

THE USE OF INTERPRETERS

I used an interpreter () it wasn't private so it did not matter

Our concern in this is the lack of communication support in essentially official and important situations for those requiring it. Of the 36 who required assistance with such communication, for two-thirds the help was usually provided by family or occasionally friends. Despite the fact that for the majority of the sample, their preferred communication involved signing (either BSL or SSE), only eight of them talked of using sign language interpreters, and this was in exceptional circumstances rather than the rule. In the interview as a whole, only 21 (34%) made any mention of interpreters, and four of these were to say that they never used them. Only six (10%) had used them more than just on very rare occasions. This confirms the findings of an earlier study, that 'The most important source of help for those requiring interpretation was the informal network of family and friends both deaf and hearing' (Sainsbury, 1986, p. 103). It should be noted that when we talk of interpreters here we include social workers, for at the time referred to in the interview, social workers often acted as interpreters and the terms tended to be used interchangeably. Current professional practice, which we would endorse, is to distinguish between these two professions and social workers are insisting that interpreting should be carried out by those expressly trained to do so.

A feature of the service provided by interpreters is that it is confidential, and this is embodied in their code of practice. Despite this, even those who had used them did not seem aware of this, some even commenting they would use interpreters when it was not private, and in private situations they would use family or friends.

I used an interpreter – else I could not go on my own, so I had an interpreter, he gave me a lift. I couldn't go on my own on the bus as I had German measles. It wasn't private, so it did not matter.
Keith, 19 years, BSL

Our concern here is threefold. Firstly, that very many of the people whose work involves interacting with the general public on a day-to-day basis had little awareness of deafness or how to communicate with a deaf person, and some (including doctors) actually seemed afraid of the situation. Secondly, that when help with communication was required, it was almost always provided by the family and that this was often in areas that are generally considered private, or where the young person should really be asserting their own independence. Thirdly, there seemed to be a general lack of awareness of interpreters and their role on the part of the deaf young people, their families, and professionals who rarely requested their services.

GETTING AROUND

He's been a lot further than I have

As will be seen in the next chapter, young deaf people often have a network of friends country wide. Often, this happened because the young deaf person had attended special school and maintained contact with friends made there. Those who attended Deaf Clubs also often made friends from other areas and visits to other Deaf Clubs were common. For the most part the deaf young people moved about, in their own locality and often around the country, with ease and confidence.

> *Oh, Paula tours the country! She does. I mean she is going to London this weekend. She was in Birmingham last weekend. She is going to Glasgow next weekend.*
> Mother of Paula, 24 years, BSL

> *I don't know. He's all over – Birmingham, Coventry. () He'll probably walk out of here and say, 'I'm going to Northampton Deaf Club', and they'll say, 'Let's go to Coventry or Birmingham or Rugby', so he could be anywhere.*
> Mother of Clive, 20 years, BSL

And, as the mother at the beginning of this section pointed out:

> *He's been a lot further than I have.*
> Mother of Bobby, 20 years, SSE

Based on the parents' reports, 18 (22%) were confident with all forms of travel, including travel by air, 42 (51%) had used both buses and planes, 19 (23%) used buses alone, and only 2 (2%) had never used public transport. However, the difficulties in using public transport experienced by all travellers, could for the deaf young person be major problems, because of the inaccessibility of information, communication difficulties at the time, or difficulties because the phone was not available to them to make contact with friends or others who could come to their aid. Parents often expressed a concern about their sons and daughters travelling around the country visiting friends, as this often involved extensive use of public transport systems.

One of the most fraught means of public transport, according to many parents of the young people, was the bus system. Almost all the young people (80, 98%) in the study had used buses alone, but many had had negative experiences. Their problems were not generally due to using bus timetables, as most (57, 70%) could follow such documents. Their difficulties were largely due to the lack of understanding shown by bus drivers and conductors, as the following quote details:

> *It's like she gets on a bus () with the right change () and she can put her money down then, like, says its 22p. 'Twenty-two' and he'll say, 'Pardon? What?' And she will say, 'Twenty-two' and she will point to it. And he's going, 'I don't understand you'. The odd times I have got on with her, you know, I will say, 'The money is there, she wants a twenty-two; if she had wanted change she wouldn't have put the two pence there'. 'Oh well, how am I supposed to know!' So she gets this all the time.*
> *Mother of Veronica, 21 years, SSE*

> *I can remember a big upset one day connected with a bus fare, when she was going to work from H... and the conductor put her off the bus. I don't think she could understand why. She has the disabled person's bus pass and she had been paying her fare. Somebody had told her how much it was and she paid the fare regularly and she had been going for weeks. Then she asked for this particular 10p or whatever it was one day and the conductor made her get off the bus and she never did understand why. You see, there again, she was on...and she rang up crying because the conductor had made her get off the bus and of course we couldn't understand what she was talking about. Tom (husband) had to get the car out and go rushing off to take her to work. But that was a sort of silly thing, she went all to pieces. I said to her afterwards, 'Why didn't you wait for the next bus and get on it?' She said she hadn't got any change, but she had used the change to ring us up! She just lost all control. But that was certainly something she didn't understand and she was embarrassed, I think, having the chap argue with her.*
> *Mother of Carol, 23 years, oral*

Independently, or with the help of their parents, many of the young people in our study prepared carefully for their bus journey, sometimes making written prompts.

> *She has got into this habit now of telling people even on a bus or anything like that, she will tell them she is deaf. I mean when they first*

started to go on a bus, I used to write it down, 'You want a 25p return'. We put 'from so and so to so and so' – just a little card for her like until she got used to going on buses.
Father of Sharon, 21 years, BSL

You see now if he goes on the bus – he goes on the bike most times, but last week he got a puncture – he went on the bus and what he does he writes the name of the road and the bus stop he wants to get off at and he always says, 'I try speech first for the road', and if the driver doesn't understand he just shows them the piece of paper. I've known him have it in his hand like that (demonstrates a piece of paper in her palm and obscured from view). You see they don't want to draw attention to themselves. Some drivers are patient and others aren't. You get that with normal people.
Mother of Shaun, 21 years, BSL

For one of the young people their worst experience had been on a bus, travelling to school.

There was a sudden blizzard. All the traffic came to a standstill. He was stuck on this bus. There must have been a loss of communication as to what was happening and nobody understood him and he couldn't understand what everybody else was doing, and they were trying to get through. Then the bus broke down. They managed to get another bus. () When he got into…there was all this snow; he walked from the bus station to the school, but he got there on foot in a blizzard, and that was his worst experience. He couldn't contact anybody.
Mother of Darren, 22 years, BSL

Travelling by train could be quite a hazardous activity for deaf people. Last-minute timetable or platform changes and unexpected delays announced over tannoy systems are not accessible to deaf people, or many hearing people, for that matter. The recent introduction of platform based visual displays of passenger information has gone some way to improve matters, though it is not a total solution, and not always to be relied on. Nearly two-thirds of the young people in our study (60/82, 73%) had used trains alone or with deaf friends and a number of these had experienced difficulties.

I prepare myself well. I check trains, etc. I check everything is all right. There are no timetables sometimes. The megaphones often tell people to change platform, but I don't know, because there is no visual display.
Phillip, 19 years, SSE

Interestingly, the apparently more complex task of travelling by air was relatively easy for the deaf young people who had travelled this way, because, designed as it is for international passengers, messages are clearly conveyed and visual displays exploited to the full. Nearly one-quarter (19/82, 23%) had travelled in planes alone or with friends.

*Mother: They are going again in three weeks' time for a fortnight. I mean, they all go. She obviously doesn't hear their announcements, I mean they have just **got** to look at the board.*

Father: I mean, I don't mess about. I just kick them out of the car and kick them their cases and go, I'm off.

Mother: We have always said like when they book in to tell them they are deaf, so they look out for them like, you know. We have always said they have got to look at the board for when their flight comes up, so they do. They've been twice now, haven't they?

Parents of Sharon, 21 years, BSL

As the instructor said, it's giving him a new challenge

The parents reported that a significant proportion (39, 48%) of the young people in our study could drive, and a further 14 (17%) were learning. It is hardly surprising that they were keen to learn, given their experiences as users of the various forms of public transport. In earlier sections of the chapter, difficulties in communicating with public officials were described, yet it is interesting to note that there was no single instance of a young person learning to drive mentioning any difficulties either in arranging lessons or communicating with the instructor. The preferred language was not a significant element here, as 22/31 (71%) BSL users, 9/13 (69%) SSE users and 21/30 (70%) of those who were oral had passed the test or were learning to drive.

We made up special signs – brake, signal – I was quite comfortable.
Ray, 21 years, oral

Interviewer: How did you communicate with your driving instructor?
Janet: I was at school when I had my lessons and my driving instructor was very...he knew what to do and he used to do all the signs and I just followed.
Interviewer: How did he come to know what to do?
Janet: Well, how come? Because other people from my school were deaf. But then I changed to a new instructor just before I had my test and I explained to him what to do, then. The same with the examiner, just explained beforehand. There was no problem.
Janet, 22 years, oral

He's learning to drive and it's going well. It's as the instructor said, it's giving him a new challenge, learning a deaf person how to drive.
Mother of Ivan, 21 years, BSL
Father: He'd never taken a deaf girl before and he says, 'How do I communicate?' I said, 'It is going to be a bit difficult, because she lip reads quite well, but obviously she can't be, driving a car. He said, 'Don't worry, I'll get something going'.
Mother: And he did. () She only had 17 lessons when he put her in for her test and she passed first go.
Parents of Sharon, 21 years, BSL

It is interesting to consider whether driving instructors are specially skilled communicators when compared to others who come into contact with deaf people, or whether the task is prescribed in such a way that it is easy to develop communication. Certainly, it is a situation where good communication is essential, and can be a matter of life and death. Our impression is that because driving instructors accepted the work, they were able to find a way to communicate.

She wouldn't hear somebody walk up behind her

Parents were concerned for the personal safety of their offspring, in particular their daughters, when they were driving or travelling alone. This was a concern not only when they were travelling, but also when they were walking at night or in secluded areas; parents felt that as the young deaf people were unlikely to hear someone walking up behind them, they were vulnerable to muggings or personal attacks.

Mother: She started cooking at D... and one side of the road it is fields and the tutor asked me to come up and find how lonely it was. It would be, up there, because Mary can't hear anybody coming up behind her with soft shoes in the dark.
()
Interviewer: And did the teacher then really think she shouldn't go?
Mother: Yes, she stopped going.
Mother of Mary, 23 years, BSL

There is so much happening and so many yobbos out there. I think what I used to worry about with Rosemary would be that she might be walking from a bus stop or something and she wouldn't hear somebody walk behind her. You know, that kind of thing.
Mother of Rosemary, 21 years, oral

I worry about all the muggings you hear about. If somebody's going to attack you, you hear somebody walking up behind you. She's still on my mind a lot, she's still my little girl.
Mother of Angela, 19 years, oral

The only problem is she wouldn't hear anybody walking behind her – you know, that happens in broad daylight, you don't have to be late at night. So if somebody was going to come up and attack her, she obviously wouldn't hear.
Mother of Sharon, 21 years, BSL

Whether or not deaf young women are in reality in more danger is difficult to ascertain. Certainly, though, for some of them their lives are affected by the feeling of greater danger either by themselves or their parents. Certainly measures that make it somewhat safer for hearing people, the ability to phone for help, or just to phone for a taxi may be more difficult. Parents took certain steps to try and protect their daughters.

The vulnerability of being deaf and coming home late at night and that sort of thing. There's an extra vulnerability of being deaf. I just made sure she had enough money and I tell her if she is in any doubt to get a taxi.
Mother of Paula, 25 years, BSL

These parents had bought their daughter a car.

Mother: We got her a car when she was seventeen and for the last year I was determined that she would be able to drive as soon as she could. () But then we worried ourselves sick. I wished we hadn't bought it then.
Father: Well if you don't worry about them going in cars, you worry about them going in trains, don't you? Janet's friends are spread all over, so it is either go in the car all over or go on the train, and on balance I think I feel happier about her going in the car than on some of these train journeys that she has to make.
Parents of Janet, 22 years, oral

Car travel was then not without its anxieties. Serious incidents involving women car-drivers who were attacked whilst trying to get assistance after breaking down had received considerable media coverage at the time of many of the interviews. Some parents felt that deafness left their sons and daughters especially vulnerable, as some of them would be unable to ask or call for help successfully, as many were unable to use a conventional telephone to alert their families or emergency services to their need for assistance. Obtaining assistance from strangers seems increasingly problematic.

Table 5.2. *Extent of use of hearing aids*

	Number	%
Always	32	55
Usually	7	12
Rarely	5	9
Never	11	19
No aid	3	5

She does drive. We do worry about the possibility of her breaking down. We do worry about her travelling.
Father of Amanda, 20 years, oral

The increasing availability of text telephones (described later in this chapter) does go some way to alleviate this problem, and gives deaf people more possibility of travelling safely. These are increasingly being installed in public places and it would seem essential that they become even more available, so that deaf people can feel free to travel around and thus participate in activities that are generally available.

THE IMPACT OF TECHNOLOGY

In the previous sections dealing with deaf young people in a hearing world, a number of issues have been identified. Firstly, the lack of public awareness about deafness; secondly, the limited access to general information for some young deaf people; and thirdly, difficulties in communication in the face-to-face situation. The first of these is a recurring theme of this book and is discussed in more detail in the final chapter. The second and third are considered further here in terms of the advances in technology, which may be relevant.

I can't manage without my hearing aid

They don't help me hear

Most people would consider hearing aids to be essential and important to young deaf people. However, the young deaf people in our study were not all enthusiastic about hearing aids. While most (95%, 55/58, three could not answer) had hearing aids, the number who actually used them was far less, as is shown in Table 5.2. Hearing aids were useful for two-thirds of the sample and little used by the other third. For convenience, in the rest of this

Table 5.3. *Use of hearing aids (young person's report) by hearing loss and by preferred language*

	Preferred language			Hearing loss		
	BSL	SSE	Oral	Profound	Severe	Moderate/ partially hearing
Always, usually	12	5	22	6	20	13
Never/rarely	11	5	3	10	5	4

section we will group those who always and those who usually wear aids together into a high-use group and those who rarely or those who never wear aids, or those who have no aid, together into a negligible-use group. All of those with no aid would never have used it anyway, and the aid was lost or discarded.

With all these categories, agreement with parents' reports is high. If the high-use group and the negligible-use group are compared with similar parent categories, they are found to be highly related, ($\chi^2 = 38.25$, $p < 0.001$). Even so, there were a few extreme discrepancies. In one case, the parents claimed the aid was worn all the time, and the young person reported it was worn rarely. In another, the young person claimed to wear it always, and the parent said it was rarely worn. However, overall agreement was high, with most errors concerning differences between 'rarely' and 'usually', rather than between the more extreme categories.

The use of hearing aids showed a relationship with both preferred language and hearing loss, themselves related factors, as is shown in Table 5.3. It appears that BSL users and SSE users were equally split as to whether or not they used their aids, but not surprisingly, the vast majority (22/25, 88%) of those who were oral tended to make great use of them. This result is statistically significant ($\chi^2 = 8.611$, $p < 0.02$). Also, the less severe the loss, the more likely the young people were to wear the hearing aid ($\chi^2 = 8.390$, $p < 0.020$), although there was a small minority with the lesser losses who did not wear them. All of these said they heard better without aids. Of those who had aids, some had always liked them, whereas some had appreciated them more as they became older.

It does help me; I can't manage without it.
Daniel, 21 years, oral

I can't manage without my hearing aid at all. I can lip read without, but I don't like not wearing my hearing aids. When I was a child, I never did. I

always wanted to wear my hearing aids; I never threw them out like
some children did.
Janet, 22 years, oral

I don't like it without them. When I was young I hated them, because
they were so bulky. When I was 14 I got post-aural aids and since then
I've always wanted to wear them.
Colin, 24 years, BSL

Sometimes their use was not for speech, but to maintain contact with the
environment.

I wear them when I go out so I am aware of cars coming and things
around me.
Veronica, 21 years, SSE

I like it for music and it makes me safer on the roads.
Jenny, 19 years, SSE

An issue for those who wanted to wear them was the greater difficulty in
getting leads and batteries, once they had left school. Supply is more or less
automatic while within the education system, but once the young person
left school the onus was on them to get leads and batteries and to arrange
repairs. Distance could be an issue, or the need to take time away from
work, as the relevant centres were only open in office hours. Possession of
'the book' (an official document, endorsing the deaf person's right to aids,
leads and batteries) was also critical. Often this had not been supplied
while they were at school, but without it many hearing-aid centres refused
to service the aids, or even supply batteries.

I'd like to wear two aids, but I like to save the batteries. It's a long way to
go and get the batteries and I can manage with only one, although it
means I can't tell the direction that sound is coming from.
Ray, 21 years, oral

You see, if I went to the hospital, if I saw this fellow, he was deaf
himself, () there was never any problem – handful of leads, handful of
batteries. But this stupid woman, she used to say, 'Where's his book?'
and I used to explain that he hadn't got a book, that he'd never had a
book, blah, blah, blah. And this went on until 18 months ago, when
finally they issued Christopher with a book.
Father of Christopher, 21 years, BSL

You have to have a book to get batteries at M… hospital, which is very
difficult. I used to go down there to get batteries or have someone look

at her hearing aid. There would be a woman doing her nails. I used to knock at the door. 'Wait a minute, have you got her book?' () You'd think they were going to give you the world. Without those batteries the hearing aids are no good.
Mother of Shirley, 22 years, SSE

This family eventually chose to go to a private centre to have ear moulds made, and to obtain the other items they required.

You try not to annoy people, because you think that maybe I shall still need them, but I don't need M...hospital. I can go to (private supplier) and can get all I want. I can be treated like a lady up there and you really are. 'Hello, Mrs P..., nice to see you again'. I go down there (the hospital) and I can queue for two hours and then they say 'Dr... has gone out on a private case'. By the time you've finished, everyone has been there for four and a half hours and some with two tots.
Mother of Shirley, 22 years, SSE

Those who did not use their aids made this choice for a number of reasons, from their being of no use, to their being noisy or intrusive or embarrassing.

Listen – nothing. Sixteen – stop aids, finish.
Diana, 20 years, BSL (gloss)

I don't wear hearing aids, I get fed up with the noises they make.
Bridget, 22 years, BSL

They get in the way, so I don't wear them now. They irritate me, and when I'm making hay they get caught up in the straw, and they make awful noises.
Geoffrey, 21 years, oral

Hearing aids give me a headache.
Zoe, 19 years, BSL

Wearing hearing aids is an indication that the person is deaf. For some this was positive but for others negative.

I never wear hearing aids, because my friends laugh at me and that makes me feel embarrassed.
Sam, 18 years, BSL

If I meet people and I'm wearing a hearing aid, it makes them shout and I don't like that.
Geoffrey, 21 years, oral

If I wear them, then people think I am stupid, or like something from outer space. People keep asking, 'What's that?'
Darren, 22 years, BSL

When I got older, I realised it didn't help. Maybe I should still wear it, though, so that people realise that I'm deaf.
Louise, 22 years, oral

Some had discarded their aids in adulthood, despite always having worn them as a child. It must be assumed these had made an informed choice based on experience, as they had had time to consider whether they were useful or not.

My teacher made me wear them when I was small, but as soon as I was old enough I took them off.
Sam, 18 years, BSL

I don't believe in them. If children don't want to wear them, they should be allowed to give them up. My mother made me wear an aid but I've given it up. The teacher said it would be good for me and my mother believed her.
Paula, 24 years, BSL

It is interesting to see how early experience of hearing aids relates to later use. We looked at those in the sample of young people who had answered the question about wearing aids and who were over three and a half at the time of the first interview study, giving a sample of 40. We looked at the age at which they received their aid, the advice that had been given at the time, the extent to which they wore the aid as a child and their attitude to it then. A comparison of this information with the extent to which they report using aids in adulthood is shown in Table 5.4.

Neither the age at which the aid was first worn, nor the adequacy of the advice given, show a significant relationship with the extent of later aid use. However, both the amount worn early on and the attitude to the aid do show a relationship with the amount of time the aid was worn at the time of the later study (amount: $\chi^2 = 6.166$, $p < 0.05$; attitude; $\chi^2 = 13.55$, $p < 0.01$). The stronger relationship is with the early attitude, and all of those who were reported as disliking their aids early on wear their aids a negligible amount now. This seems to indicate that some children, even if encouraged to wear aids, never do come to accept them.

We were interested to discover that most of the young people felt that deaf children should be made to wear hearing aids. Of the 49 who could answer the question, only four (8%) thought children should be free to

Table 5.4. *Early experience and later use of hearing aids*

	Always/usually	Rarely/never
Age aids obtained		
Before 12 months	2	0
At 13–24 months	8	7
At 25 + months	13	10
Advice given when a child		
Adequate	14	9
Minimal	8	5
None	1	3
Amount worn as a child		
All day	17	6
Sometimes	5	10
Never	1	1
Attitude to aid as a child		
Tolerated	16	6
Varied	7	3
Disliked	0	8

choose, with nearly two-thirds (30, 61%) thinking they should be made to wear them. The remainder (15/49, 31%) thought it depended on the child or on the situation. There was not a significant relationship between whether the young person wore their aids and whether they thought that children should be made to.

> *Young person who wears aid: Children, yes, well, it depends whether they've got some hearing or not. If they're profoundly deaf, it's really not worth it. If they are severely or partially deaf, yes, they should wear hearing aids. It depends what hearing they've got.*
> *Young person who does not wear aid: Yes, I really think they should, because it will make them hear. If they don't wear hearing aids they will become spoilt. They must use hearing aids.*

Once teletext came along it made such a difference

The most widely used piece of equipment, not surprisingly, was teletext TV, and two-thirds (54, 66%) had it available to them. This allows subtitles to be superimposed on some television programmes, although it is not available for all programmes. Without subtitles, watching television could be disruptive for hearing members of a family, as many of the deaf young people would request explanations and clarifications.

> *The thing is, when I am watching telly he says, 'What did they say?' and you have missed the next bit. That is the thing that gets me down.*
> *Mother of Gavin, 19 years, oral*

This family found teletext a real boon for precisely that reason.

> *He loves television. . .and all our viewing was interrupted by explaining to Colin what was happening and by the time we had explained we had lost track of the programme. We used to get frustrated, Colin used to get frustrated and it was a vicious circle. But once teletext came along it made such a difference that we could follow the programmes.*
> *Mother of Colin, 24 years, BSL*

> *Mother: She has got a teletext we bought her just before Christmas. ()*
> *Interviewer: Does she like it?*
> *Mother: She is over the moon.*
> *Father: We wish we had got it before now.*
> *Mother: It is making so much difference. I am astonished to listen to her. She watches the news, she is interested in. . .She said to me on the phone last night, 'Did you watch Antiques Roadshow?' and I said, 'No I didn't', and she said, 'It was fantastic, I was so thrilled with it' and I thought, 'How marvellous' and she has missed all of this all of this time.*
> *Parents of Carol, 23 years, oral*

As young people gain access to television through subtitles, those programmes that are not subtitled are all the more frustrating.

> *They don't do enough (subtitling). Neighbours – at the moment she is really going mad with waiting for that to be done. You know, there aren't enough programmes on. Because it is very frustrating for all of us, well say for me and her, because when she watches Neighbours I have to sit down and watch it with her and tell her everything that has been said and I have no time to listen. Trying to listen what they said and trying to tell her at the same time – a bit difficult, you know.*
> *Mother of Rosemary, 21 years, oral*

Since this interview, Neighbours has been subtitled.

Most of the families without teletext described the cost as prohibitive.

> *We don't have teletext in this house. They (his parents) say it is not worth it, because it is too much money.*
> *Michael, 20 years, oral*

Interestingly, there were rare instances where teletext was available but the young people chose not to use it.

I prefer to watch without subtitles. Sometimes you are watching the subtitles and you're missing the picture. So I prefer to watch it without subtitles, and listen to the sound. I have a TV link, a microphone that takes the sound straight into the ear.
Trevor, 22 years, oral

A further example is discussed in Chapter 7.

By chance, one of the group discussions took place one week after Deaf Awareness Event on Channel 4, where a full day was fully subtitled and interpreted into sign language. The young people enjoyed the access afforded by this, but raised some interesting points. Firstly, it was much more relaxing with everything interpreted; they could come and go as they pleased instead of having to be there for a particular time.

Paula: You look at it totally differently. I didn't watch it all the way through. I just used it as a break. We were sitting down after work, you know. Normally, if you stick the television on, then there are lots of problems, things on the news that you can't follow that are sort of boring. I was really relaxed that day with Channel 4, had a cup of tea and, say, watched it for half an hour and then got ready to cook or whatever, just the same as hearing people do.

Secondly, they particularly enjoyed the advertisements and found them very entertaining. Thirdly and possibly most importantly, they appreciated the incidental information provided, and had not realised that hearing people had this available to them as a matter of course.

Paula: I found it interesting – the bit before the programme started, they said, 'This programme is Children of a Lesser God; it is about deaf relationships'. There was always sort of a little advertisement that's normally the information that deaf people miss and hearing people get.
Carol: Yes, my husband recorded that; I heard the information and then they were talking about the deaf actress at the end. I never realised they talked about the film afterwards. ( ) On ITV they had the interpreter talking about what was happening on the other side, what was happening on the other stations; that was really interesting.
Paula: She was sort of saying what else was on later in the week and normally hearing people know what's on next or what's on later. It was much better having the interpreter telling us the same. I wish it was always on, so we got the information too.

While it is unlikely that on-screen interpretation will ever be available for more than a minority of programmes, the importance of subtitling should not be underestimated. Access to television is significant for a number of reasons, including entertainment. However, its potential as a source of general information, cultural as well as factual, is probably of the greatest significance. Soap operas, as well as the news and documentary programmes, convey information on such matters as mortgages or getting into debt. While the accuracy of life as portrayed in soap operas is a matter for debate, they often portray situations where issues are not clear cut and where there are dilemmas without simple solutions. Some families also saw television as assisting and developing English skills:

> *Apart from anything else, it helps to educate the children, because they read and they get the language flow from it. The deaf think in a different way. They only use words that are necessary. () When they write anything on paper, they write in a back-to-front sort of way. And teletext makes so much difference.*
> *Mother of Colin, 24 years, BSL*

The extent of subtitling is increasing all the time. From 30 minutes in 1980, BBC TV in 1992 was subtitling 44 hours a week, with ITV 15 hours a week and Channel 4 20 hours a week, overall between 9% and 29% of total output. The Broadcasting Act of 1990 requires that at least half of Channel 3 and Channel 5 programmes are subtitled and Channel 4 has voluntarily agreed to this. This is partly in response to pressure from the Deaf Broadcasting Campaign.

After teletext, the next most popular aid was the vibrating alarm. These are alarms that are placed under the sleeper's pillow and vibrate, instead of emitting sound, at a preset time. Nearly two-thirds (49, 60%) of the young people in our sample had non-auditory alarms designed especially for deaf people.

> *He has got one of those (vibrating pillow). () Oh gosh, life would be impossible without. He would be late every day.*
> *Mother of Colin, 24 years, BSL*

Without such alarms, they were often dependent on others to wake them up.

> *It interferes with us. When he's going out at 5 o'clock in the morning, the van comes for him at 6 o'clock. He's not got an alarm pillow. I often wonder how he used to manage when he wasn't with us. () Its like the parent–child relationship still, that sort of thing.*
> *Mother of Darren, 22 years, BSL*

And not all found vibrating alarms to be that successful.

*Like if he starts work at 6 a.m. we have to wake him at 4.30 a.m. He's
got a pillow, a vibrating pillow, but it's no good. So we have to wake
him. It's things like that we need to do. He's 23 and we still have to do it.*
Father of Anil, 23 years, BSL

*Even getting up in the morning is the biggest job of their life. It's going to
work, it's getting up. They've got a vibrator alarm, but they don't sleep
on them. They move, you see. It's like a bar of soap. It slips up by the
pillow and ends up on the floor. I go up every morning and turn it off.
It's on the floor. We have to get them up for work. It is a full-time job.
She relies we're going to get them up.*
Father of Shirley, 22 years, SSE

This situation of young people living away from home who still relied on
their parent to wake them up was not unique, and we were told of at least
three instances. Having to depend on someone else to wake them up denied
those without adapted alarms an important aspect of independence and
contributed to an overall high degree of dependence on parents in this
aspect of their lives. This issue is discussed further in Chapter 9.

One further set of auditory systems devised for hearing people are baby
alarms. These systems depend on the user being able to hear bells, bleepers
or amplified sounds. Only three of the young people in the study were
parents and only two of these actually lived in the same home as their child
or children. Of these two, only one was unable to hear a conventional baby
alarm. This young woman was married to a deaf man and as such they
needed an adapted non-auditory baby alarm. The alarm flashed when their
baby cried and thus they were alerted to the baby's cries.

Finally, a further auditory system found widely in the average home is a
doorbell or buzzer. For the most part the young deaf people in our sample
were felt by parents to be unable to hear a knock on their door or the sound
of a door bell. The majority of these, however, depended upon other
members of their family to respond to callers. Only a quarter (20, 24%) of
the young people made use of specially adapted doorbells attached to the
electric light system in their homes. When doorbells were rung with this
system in operation, the lights in certain rooms of the house would flash on
and off, thus alerting members of the household to the presence of a caller.
While the absence of these was generally because they were not thought to
be important, or they were too difficult to obtain, one family had
deliberately not had these fitted.

*There are two ways of looking at that, actually. I prefer them, if
somebody knocked on the door, I would prefer them not to go anyway,*

if they were on their own. If we were here, we would answer it. If they were on their own, I would prefer they didn't answer it anyway – security, I suppose. You don't know who is at the door these days, do you?

Father of Sharon and her deaf sibling, 21 years, BSL

A further aid available was the text telephone, and 15 (18%) had these available. However, the telephone was a more significant part of these deaf young people's lives than this would indicate, as we discuss in the next section.

THE TELEPHONE

She uses the telephone as a signal

In Chapter 4 we described how an inability to use the telephone was often cited by parents as one cause of lack of job progression in the working lives of the young deaf people. Despite the fact that many of the young people could not use the telephone in conventional ways, with consequences for their personal and social lives, it nevertheless featured in the lives of most of them.

When we examined the current use made of telephones by the young people it emerged that, despite their hearing loss and the limited availability of text telephones, only just over a third (30, 37%) had never used a telephone at all, according to their parents. A further four (5%) of the young people used text telephone systems only, although more than this number had access to them. Only seven (9%) could converse on an unadapted telephone, with a further 13 (16%) being able to converse using a telephone amplifier.

> *Mother: I mean, he's got ever so good and he does make mistakes, but I can say that he can use the telephone and he rings to tell us what time to meet him, etc.*
> *Father: Yes, and he does phone his friends.*
> *Parents of David, 20 years, oral*

> *We have had an amplifier fitted on to that (points to phone) and we find he can talk to his mates as long as he knows who is on the other end, because again it is a little bit of guesswork.*
> *Mother of Wayne, 21 years, oral*

The young people themselves also talked of the guesswork involved.

I can use the telephone. I understand about one word in three and I can usually manage.
Jeremy, 20 years, oral

And parents described the systems adopted by the young people.

She'll phone the shop and she will phrase the question so the answer is a 'yes' or a 'no'. She can use it in an emergency to give a message.
Mother of Tina, 18 years, oral

This could be stressful, however.

With men, they've got lower voices, I can hear them with no bother. With women speaking to me, I have difficulty hearing. Higher voices I can't hear very well on the phone.
Interviewer: How do you manage when you have women on the phone?
I tell them, I have to make an excuse, I say, 'The line's bad, can you speak up, please'. Also, I find women speak a lot quicker than men do; they talk faster, mumbo jumbo. () I get frightened, now and again. People that don't know I'm deaf and that. They talk to me, they...like when I'm talking to somebody on the phone and they don't explain and they keep going on and on, and they don't help you. That's when I get mad.
Trevor, 22 years, oral

More ingeniously, a further ten (12%) used the telephone to speak, understanding very simple responses like 'yes' and 'no'.

I will do the talking. Mum will say just 'yes' when she understands. I know the phone is answered because of the change in tone.
Ray, 21 years, oral

I can tell if its my mother or father on the phone. I talk to them. I can't ask questions or hear them talk. We have a code: 'Yes, Zoe' for yes, two words; and 'No' for no, one word.
Zoe, 19 years, BSL

Even some of those who could not hear any response at all made use of the phone. Eighteen (22%) used the telephone to convey verbal messages only (for example, to indicate to parents or friends that they had reached a particular destination).

I can hear the pips stop and then I talk I don't hear anything back, though.
Gavin, 19 years, oral

He can use the telephone. This is amazing, because when he comes home, if he is earlier than we expect him to be, he picks up the phone. He uses it and he can tell when we answer, because all he says is, 'Hello, bye-bye Robert', so I know he is at the station. That is for me to know that he is at the station, because he can't hear me speak, but he automatically knows when you answer, which is very good.
Mother of Robert, 22 years, BSL

*When he has been home for the weekend and he has gone back to D...,
when he arrives at D... Station he would always ring us and say that he was at D... Station and was waiting for the bus.*
Interviewer: And if you spoke?
He couldn't hear me. And sometimes he did that as well: if he got to the station here, he would telephone and say 'I am at...station, please fetch me'. We would just dash down the station and pick him up.
Mother of Christopher, 21 years, BSL

He just says when he goes out, because he drives. When he first used to go out, we used to say, 'Phone us to let us know you arrived safely'. So he used to phone and say, 'I'm all right, I'm here – fine'. But he can't hear us.
Father of Phillip, 19 years, SSE

She uses the telephone as a signal. She can give her side of the conversation to you but she can't hear what people say to her.
Mother of Angela, 19 years, oral

For one or two, desperation had lead to its use.

Sam has used the phone three times, twice when we were burgled, and once before, only when he needed help.
Father of Sam, 18 years, BSL

It is important to note that these figures relate to usage at the time of the interviews and not to potential usage; the majority of the young people would have been able to use visual telephone systems had they been available to them.

An inability to keep in touch by phone caused some parents to be particularly concerned. For one mother whose son was about to move into a home of his own, the complications of keeping in touch without a telephone seemed considerable.

That is the stomach-churning bit, because I can't phone him and he can't phone me. He has got a super neighbour who, as soon as she realised the problem, said, 'If Colin has got any problems and he wants

*to contact you he can come to me and I will phone for you and if you
need to get any message to Colin phone me'.*
Mother of Colin, 24 years, BSL

Another whose daughter lived at home noted:

*The complications that it (inability to use the phone) can give to your
life are just not appreciated. If I am away or if I am in town – I work in
town – and I am going to be late and Paula is expecting me home, I can't
let her know.*
Mother of Paula, 24 years, BSL

THE AVAILABILITY OF AIDS AND EQUIPMENT

We had to pay for it

For the most part, the young people made interesting and resourceful use
of available equipment. It was thus disappointing to realise the extent to
which it was not fully available, or information about it difficult to obtain.
As has already been mentioned, not all television programmes were
subtitled. Text telephones are now gradually becoming more widespread.
Currently more and more public and commercial companies are installing
them, allowing deaf people greater possibilities of managing their own
affairs. The time when they are installed in significant numbers of public
buildings as in some other countries is eagerly awaited.

The extract from the following interview explains some of the difficulties in getting equipment. The financial implications are apparent from
these extracts from the interview with Colin's mother, who in two earlier
quotes has described the importance of teletext for Colin.

*We've got that (flashing light doorbell). We had to pay for it and that is
another thing that is given, but we have to pay for it. They just came and
said, 'You can afford it' so we had to pay for it. For Colin's 21st we
bought him a television set of his own, with teletext, but we are in a
position to do it. Obviously we had to give something up to get that for
Colin, but a lot of parents can't do it and it's a tragedy. There are many
people who can't afford these things so they can't have them, and it
makes such a difference to our lives. And I think its a total tragedy that
they don't get it through the National Health, because there is so much
given for the blind, but the deaf get nothing.*
Mother of Colin, 24 years, BSL

The other issue for many parents was that items had to be obtained through Social Services.

We've never had any call for social work up to now. () I mean, we might have to start using social workers now he is back home, you see, for different things like servicing his hearing aids.
Mother of Shaun, 21 years, BSL

COPING WITH THE HEARING WORLD

In some situations, the young deaf people were at a disadvantage coping with the hearing world. Both difficulties in communicating and lack of access to formal and informal information contributed to this. However, in many instances, it seemed to be the attitudes of hearing people rather than the deafness itself that was the crucial factor. Many barriers could be overcome, if people had the will to do so, yet even the simplest situation could be made difficult by an unsympathetic approach. A consequence of some of these difficulties was a greater reliance on parents for some things, than might be expected of hearing young people of the same age. In health and finance, where independence is usually asserted by young people, often parents were involved. Yet in travelling in this country and abroad, and in driving themselves about, most of the young people were competent to manage matters themselves. Technological aids have a part to play. It seems ridiculous that batteries for essential equipment such as hearing aids could be difficult to obtain. Hearing aids are as significant a factor in facilitating access for deaf people, as ramps and lifts are to wheelchair users. Moreover, if deaf people are to enjoy equal rights and equal access, text telephones and subtitling needs to be made as widely available as possible.

CHAPTER SIX

Friendships, relationships and social life

I have no friends round here. I stay at home by myself. I talk to myself, I am more calm and peaceful without people.
Christopher, 21 years, BSL

Jane has been her friend since she was 12 years old. She still writes to most of her friends from being in junior school. She is still in contact with a lot of friends from D... school. They still visit. There is someone in America she writes to, and someone in Australia. She makes friends wherever she goes.
Mother of Amanda, 20 years, SSE

In the last three chapters we have considered the young people in the public worlds of school, college, work and the general public domain. We now move back into a more private sphere, that of friendships and personal relationships, and look at the social life of the young people. As we look at this topic, a complex picture emerges. Firstly, it is clear that some of the young deaf people enjoyed a rich and varied social life, often involving them in travel all over the country. On the other hand, it emerged that some were extremely lonely at times, felt isolated and had difficulty in making friends and sustaining friendships.

Table 6.1 sets out the friendship pattern of the young people as described by the parents and the young people, combining information obtained from a number of questions in each interview. The use of the category 'no friends' was very strictly applied and only used in the absence of evidence of any social contacts at all. Three sets of figures are given. The first column shows the friendship patterns of the young people based on information from their parents. The second shows the same based on

Table 6.1. *The friendship patterns of the young people*

	Parent interview		Young person interview		Parent interview (young people sample)	
	Number	%	Number	%	Number	%
Stable group of friends	39	48	30	49	32	52
Special friend	8	10	17	28	7	11
Variable, or casual friends only	25	30	12	20	18	30
No friends	5	6	1	2	0	0
Not possible to assess	5	6	1	2	4	7
Total	82		61		61	

reports of the young people. The third shows the parent reports only for those who were interviewed as young people. It is thus directly comparable with the second column.

It is interesting to note that none of those perceived by the parents as having no friends were involved in the young people interviews. Four of these had limited communication skills and one refused to be interviewed. The young person, who saw himself as having no friends, was perceived by his mother as somewhat of a loner, but as having had friends at college.

Overall, a positive pattern emerges with the majority of the sample (young people's report 77%, parents' report 57%) having a special friend or a stable group of friends, with young people more likely to report this than parents. However, the parents and the young people differed in the way in which friendship patterns were described. While there was general agreement over who was part of a stable group of friends, more young people than parents saw themselves as having a special friend, whereas more parents saw their sons and daughters as having changing friends and casual relationships only.

In the interviews, the parents of the young people tended to focus on the problems that they felt their sons and daughters had in their social lives, whereas the young people themselves presented a more positive picture. For example, 39 (64%) of the young people described themselves as seeing their friends often, and a further 19 (31%) as seeing them sometimes. Overall, they felt themselves to be in regular contact and conveyed a generally positive view. However, the parents seemed conscious of many more problems. They described 36 (44%) of the young people as having great difficulty in making friends, a further 30 (37%) as having some difficulty, with only 16 (20%) as making friends easily. This discrepancy may be because the young people saw things differently, or because they chose not to elaborate on their difficulties. Alternatively, it may be that the parents had a more conventional understanding of friendship patterns and a different view of what constituted a good social life. In this chapter, we attempt to describe in some detail the social life of the young people and to examine these paradoxes further.

MEETING AND MAKING FRIENDS

For most hearing young people, many of their friends in adult life come through continuing school relationships, from friends made at work or college, leisure activities and casual social contacts. For deaf young people, it could be expected to be the same, although for some of them, their informal contacts include friends made through Deaf Clubs. We shall examine these in turn to consider the contribution they make.

He tends to keep his friends from school

For most young hearing people, their friends in the period immediately after leaving school are those they have made at school. School, home and work are usually in the same locality, and thus school friends are still around, and they are likely to be gradually added to or changed by new friends from work or college.

For many of the young deaf people, it was different. The majority in the research sample had spent most of their school lives in some form of special educational provision, and at the secondary stage, 33 (40%) were at boarding school. For many of them, this meant that school was in a different locality from their parental home, and their own home in the post-school years. Some argue that attendance at special school provides opportunities to meet similar youngsters and establish friendships far and wide, while others see the distance between home and school as being a problem. Advocates of integration in education suggest that the develop-ment of local friends is a strong supportive argument. Others, however, see deaf children as not fitting into hearing schools and thus not making friends. We shall discuss this later in the chapter when we look at friendship patterns at school. For the moment we shall look at the persistence of school friendships into adult life.

Although, as was described in Chapter 3, some of the young people were upset to leave school and missed the regular contact with their friends, most of the young people were reported by their parents as still seeing friends from school, 30 (37%) regularly and 37 (45%) occasionally. The young people were not asked specifically how often they saw their school friends.

The close friends she's got she's had most of her life. They are her school friends. She's got more deaf friends than hearing friends. She just sees her friends at weekends. I do think she is a bit lonely. She lives on her own. I do think it is a lonely disability.
Mother of Samantha, 21 years, BSL, School for the Deaf until 11 years, then PHU

Well, Pam she really knows. Pam and Tracey, like. You know, because they have all been to school together, like, they tend to stick together.
Interviewer: They stick together? Do they meet at Deaf Club?
Yes, or she goes round their house like Thursday nights and they will go out Saturdays and Sundays.
Mother of Sharon, 21 years, BSL, PHU until 11 years, then boarding at school for the deaf

He has always kept this group of hearing friends locally at the end of the road, because he wasn't a boarder. Probably because he played with them before he left school. They didn't go to his school, because they were all normal, you see. He would play with them at night time, cricket and football on the rec, and go train spotting with them, you see.
Mother of Wayne, 21 years, oral, day pupil at school for the deaf throughout

He tends to keep his friends from school. () He's been abroad three times with an old school friend. () He has a group of friends, not just one best friend. He goes out Fridays, certainly weekends. Goes to the pub, a disco sometimes and then football sometimes.
Mother of John, 22 years, oral, mainstream school throughout

The quotes above confirm that going away to school did not necessarily create problems for later social life. However, some parents felt that going to a school outside the locality had meant that friendships were more difficult to sustain after leaving school.

She had a lot of friends when she was younger, yes. But now, you see, as always happens, people go their own way. Isabel went away to school, so she lost a lot of contact with them. And of course when she went back to L... they had all made other friends and gone their own way and Isabel was more or less left. But I suppose that happens to any child that goes away to school, for whatever reason...
Mother of Isabel, 21 years, SSE

Table 6.2. *Secondary school attended and maintenance of contact with school friends – parents' account*

	School for deaf, boarding	School for deaf, non-boarding	PHU	Mainstream
Regularly	11	3	11	4
Occasionally	16	7	8	6
Never/no school friends	6	2	4	1

Note: That the total was 79, as three were at alternative special schools.

> *She was at...(boarding school). Well, now she's at...(a local college) and comes home. She hasn't got friends in the immediate neighbourhood. That means she is sometimes on her own.*
> *Father of Janet, 22 years, oral*

It seemed that, however, the other side to this was the wider network of friends that some of them established. A contrast to the view put by Janet's father above, and an illustration of the discrepancy of parent's and young people's accounts was provided by Janet's comments, talking about her friends when she was interviewed.

> *I have one in A..., who I still phone up, and I have one here in B... and she was in the bed next to me all through school, in the dormitories, and so I see a lot of her now...She is coming for Easter, and I see her once a week definitely, and sometimes twice, but she sometimes comes and stays with me overnight.*
> *Interviewer: What do you do together when you go out?*
> *Well, she is very busy and I am busy as well, so it is quite difficult, but on Wednesday nights we go to the Deaf Club round here, and that is good. Last week with some other friends from Deaf Club we went for a meal. We went to a night club, I think. Weekends if I'm free, I go over to her house, maybe for the day, have lunch.*
> *Janet, 22 years, oral*

It seems that here Janet, with justification, saw her social life as rich, whereas her father was aware of the times she spent at home when compared to her hearing sister.

There was in fact, no difference in whether or not the young people retained friends from school and the type of school attended (see Table 6.2) although of course the way in which the contact was maintained could be different.

Table 6.3. *Friends at work and college –*
parents' account

	Number	%
Work		
Yes, meets outside	20	32
Yes, but at work only	19	30
No	23	37
Not known	1	2
College		
Yes, meets outside	18	32
Yes, but at work only	20	35
No	18	32
Not known	1	2

Therefore, the vast majority of the young people, regardless of type of school attended, continued to see school friends, after they had left school. In all categories except PHUs the contact was more likely to be occasional rather than regular, but none of the differences are statistically significant.

She's made friends at work but it hasn't gone on from there

Conventionally, one's place of work provides a source of potential friends. Most (63, 77%) of the young deaf people at the time of the interviews were in some form of work (we shall include for this analysis, permanent jobs, job schemes and sheltered workshops). However, as Table 6.3 indicates, whilst nearly two thirds of these (39/63, 62%) were felt to have made friends at work, almost half (19/39, 49%) of these friendships were confined to the workplace only, that is to say that work friends were not met out of working hours. A similar picture also emerged for college, as is also shown in Table 6.3.

At work they're a bit older – they don't want to know. They've got their own life and they're not interested in taking him out.
Mother of Ivan, 21 years, BSL

She's made friends at work, but it hasn't gone on from there. She doesn't get invited to anybody's birthday or night out or anything.
Mother of Jean, 22 years, SSE

Interviewer: What about work – is there anybody he meets out of work?
No – well, there is one he has seen. He doesn't go out with them, does he?
Mother of Wayne, 21 years, oral

To some extent this lack of contact out of working hours can be explained, as it would be for hearing people, in terms of lack of shared interests and so on. Parents, however, proffered a number of additional explanations; some focused on the difficulties deaf people have in carrying on conversations at the same time as doing their work.

His work is involved with hearing people, but you see, you put a deaf person working at a bench and there is no conversation. Whereas hearing people can talk as they are working, he can't.
Mother of Robert, 22 years, BSL

Where the others can sit and natter to each other, she can't; she has to get on with her work, because she can't work and listen at the same time.
Mother of Isabel, 21 years, SSE

Parents also described the reluctance their sons and daughters felt to join groups of hearing people because of the high likelihood of their being excluded, no matter how good the intentions of their colleagues.

*He doesn't socialise with them. He has to be doing something **with** hearing people. He can't just go out for a chat. He copes very well, but with the majority of hearing people he has difficulty having an in-depth conversation. He got on well with his fellow students and a lot of his close friends regret that they couldn't get closer to Ray, but it was because of the deafness.*
Mother of Ray, 21 years, oral

Even when friends were seen outside work, it was for more formal, rather than casual events.

He has got his friends at work, so he gets invited occasionally to parties with the friends at work who I think just invite him. It is not that he mixes very well with people, but he goes to 21st and engagement parties and things like that.
Mother of Colin, 24 years, BSL

Interviewer: So she goes out with the girls from work.
Oh yes, they have makeup parties, she went to a wedding, she goes out Christmas with them.
Mother of Sharon, 21 years, BSL

This could include attending celebrations for the deaf young person.

I think that (21st) was one of the best times for us () and he had a wonderful time. I was worried to death, but there were a lot of hearing

people there; there were a lot of deaf people there. His work mates came
– great bunch of fellows. They even arranged a kiss-o-gram for him!
You know, it was so normal.
Mother of Colin, 24 years, BSL

These quotes are interesting, because, although they indicate positive
relationships at work, they were often not so much casual informal
relationships, but focused around structured formal events. Some parents
made this point explicitly. The remark that when with hearing people the
deaf young people had to be 'doing something' was echoed by a number of
parents. It did seem that when the young people were invited out it was to
more structured social occasions; for the young women, frequent mention
was made of invitations to engagement parties, weddings and make-up
parties, whereas the young men were invited to darts matches and snooker
games. Get-togethers of an unstructured kind were probably more difficult
to become involved in for the young people, as the procedures were less
predictable and would inevitably involve more verbal negotiation; a
wedding or a sports match has its own prescribed rules and deaf people can
follow established protocol. In less formal get-togethers it is not so easy to
follow the crowd or rely on remembered routine. It may well be that
hearing colleagues at work did have good intentions, and used formal
occasions to demonstrate a warmth of feeling that they could not sustain in
more informal events. The following quote shows that the young person
could be well aware of this.

She had her 21st birthday while she was at B... and they made a
tremendous thing of it. Because it was not long after that she was
screaming at me that everybody hated her. Nobody liked her, and that
sort of thing. And I said, I have never heard such rubbish'. I said, 'If they
don't like you, why on earth did they go to all that trouble over your
birthday?' because they decorated her desk and everything. It was
beautiful. It was really lovely, she was thrilled to bits and she had lovely
presents and a few weeks later she is screaming that nobody likes her.
Mother of Carol, 23 years, oral

A disturbing point, though, is that around one-third were considered by
their parents to have no friends at work and college, even if confined to
socialising in the workplace or at college only. It is apparent that some of
the young people were isolated.

It was very bad () she loved the work, she would sit at the table with the
girls she was working with and they just continued their own conver-
sation, but never included her in the conversation, even though they

spoke to her in the office and they knew that she understood them, but they never bothered to include her and that made her very unhappy and she used to go back from lunch in tears. And she said that is the problem with all her deaf friends who have jobs – they feel left out at work.
Mother of Rosemary, 21 years, oral

He hasn't got any special friends (at work) – he brought two home from the garage and he repaired cars for them, but they don't talk and once they had got their cars repaired, they had gone. You know what I mean.
Mother of Andrew, 21 years, BSL

As was mentioned in Chapter 4, some also felt talked about in the work situation, and a minority were teased.

We have included very few quotes from the young people themselves in this section, because they only very rarely mentioned work in the context of social relationships. They seemed largely to perceive work, not as a social activity, but as a means of earning money.

With hearing people it's no good, we can't cope

The difficulties described in the work situation were probably influential too in informal hearing settings for many of the young deaf people. Spoken communication in groups has already been described as problematic in the context of the family. For deaf young people with hearing friends the group situation could be difficult. At the beginning of Chapter 1, Isabel described her frustration when she had to ask her hearing boyfriend what had been said when they were together in a group of hearing people. She also commented:

With hearing people, it's no good, we can't cope. There are communication problems. It may be OK when a couple are on their own, but if in a group, say in a pub, it's no good.
Isabel, 21 years, SSE

Parents too were conscious of this difficulty.

She was willing to be friendly with everybody, but you see, she is lost in a group; she can't see what people are saying in groups, so all little parties and things they went to, she missed out; she was a bit lost there.
Mother of Janet, 22 years, oral

The only time she would feel lonely is when she was in a group of hearing people. That would be the only time, I think'.
Mother of Rosemary, 21 years, oral

I think whenever they go to the pub. He is all right if he just stays in his one little group, but if different people come and join the group then he does get a bit lost when two or three conversations start going on, the one group.
Mother of Nigel, 19 years, oral

Some of the young people attempted to explain to their friends how best to communicate and to suggest how they felt isolated when they could not follow everything, no matter how irrelevant the particular part of the conversation might seem to the hearing participants.

If I don't understand what people say, my feelings are hurt, I ask them to write it down, so I can understand too.
Andrew, 21 years, BSL

Interviewer: Do you get angry when hearing people talk and you don't understand what they are saying?
I try not to. I accept it, but I don't like it when there are two people talking across me and I say, 'What did you say?' 'Oh, nothing important'. That drives me mad.
Interviewer: So what do you do when that happens?
I say, 'Well, it might matter to me' or 'It might be important' or sometimes if I am at ease with them, I say, 'Oh well, I would like to know anyway, tell me'. Sometimes they say, 'Sorry, I didn't realise'.
Janet, 22 years, oral

For the 34 of the young people interviewed, who included hearing people among their friends and could answer the question, 19 said they had great difficulty in the group situation, five had some difficulty and only ten could converse easily.

With deaf people, I know I am with my own people

For the reasons discussed above, some of the young people were more likely to find all or some of their social life with other deaf people.

I have lots of hearing friends and I see my deaf friends at a different time. I can't really relax at work, but with deaf people I know I am with my own people.
Veronica, 21 years, SSE

Parents identified the Deaf Club as a place where communication could be relaxed and easy.

Well, I think they are very relaxed together at the Deaf Club. They all have the same disability, therefore communication is never a problem.

They're always very relaxed and happy when they are all together.
Mother of Josie, 24 years, BSL

Even when the parents had worked hard in developing the young person's spoken communication, as they felt this would provide them with greater opportunities to make friends in adult life, it did not always work out that way.

Father: I think, a point we haven't made yet, that at the back of our minds in wanting her to have an ordinary education in an ordinary environment and as a normal child, we realised she would have to live in the normal hearing world and therefore we wanted to try, as far as we were able, to keep her in it so she would not be isolated and have to live for ever in the Deaf Club, if you like, and nowhere else.
()
Mother: We always hoped she would have a social life outside the Deaf Club, but she hasn't.
Parents of Carol, 23 years, oral

Deaf Clubs were often used as meeting points, as even without fixing a meeting in advance they could feel sure of seeing people they knew.

They have always said, 'You know where the Deaf Club is; you know where we are on Wednesday nights or any time!'
Mother of Robert, 22 years, BSL

As was mentioned in the previous chapter, and in the quote that heads this chapter, many of the deaf young people travelled widely to meet their friends.

Sharon, when she gets boyfriends, they live so far away. One at Ipswich, one in Hertfordshire, one in London, one the other side of London. () They go to Coventry, they go to Crystal Palace, they go to Birmingham, they go to the one here, they have been to Luton, doing the rounds. They went to Minehead.
Mother of Sharon, 21 years, BSL

They go to Derby, Nottingham, Leicester, Birmingham, you name it, they go there. Just for a disco, just to meet different people to get the news. This is the news from Birmingham, sort of thing.
Father of Shirley, 22 years, SSE

For many of the young people, an advantage of being deaf was the feeling they belonged to a group throughout the country, and for some throughout the world.

However, not all the young people attended Deaf Clubs. One of the criticisms of Deaf Clubs that we encountered quite frequently was that many Deaf Clubs seemd to cater for an older age group who would not relinquish their hold on the organisational aspects of the Club. Also, for oral deaf young people it could be difficult to integrate into a Deaf Club, as the language used in the clubs is BSL and some are not welcoming to oral deaf people.

I don't go to Deaf Club because I don't understand the sign language and their talking confuses me. It's all right for them, though, but I don't understand, they don't use voice.
Daniel, 21 years, oral

Some had been discouraged from attending Deaf Clubs by their schools.

Never, we were not allowed (to go to Deaf Club). If I stayed with a friend who lives half way between here and the local Deaf Club I would go. But if I was at school I couldn't go.
Isabel, 21 years, SSE

For other young people, however, it was the parents who were reluctant for them to attend. There is of course a real issue here for parents, for this membership of the Deaf Club may seem to be the beginning of their son or daughter moving away from them, not in the usual adolescent way of establishing a new life, where the parents assume a different but known role, but moving into a world that is unknown, unpredictable and inaccessible.

It's a kind of community really. They are a community of their own. They don't need us.
Father of Sharon, 21 years, BSL

DEAF AND HEARING FRIENDS

Table 6.4 shows the friendship pattern of the young people as reported by their parents and the 60 young people who answered the question. As can be seen from comparing the two percentage columns, there is some inconsistency, with the young people themselves indicating their friends were either all deaf or all hearing, whereas the parents emphasised the 'mostly deaf' or 'mostly hearing' categories. This difference could not be accounted for by the different samples involved. Detailed inspection of the data showed that the major disagreements were between 'mostly' and 'all',

Table 6.4. *The friendships of the young people*

	Parents' report		Young people's report	
	Number	%	Number	%
Equal mix of deaf and hearing	11	13	7	12
Mostly deaf	34	41	7	12
All deaf	4	5	21	35
Mostly hearing	16	20	1	2
All hearing	12	15	23	38
No friends	5	6	1	2

Table 6.5. *Preferred communication and friendship pattern*

	BSL	SSE	Oral	LLS
Equal deaf and hearing	4	4	3	0
All/mostly deaf	23	8	5	2
All/mostly hearing	3	1	22	2
No friends	1	0	0	4

rather than more substantive differences. This seems to us a further indication of differences in perception of what constituted a friendship by young people and parents. However, a further factor seemed to operate here. The young people, in discussing their friends, seemed to concentrate on a much smaller group of people across a much narrower time scale, essentially talking about the friends they had here and now while the parents viewed friendships in a broader perspective. In our further analysis, we have decided to group 'all' and 'mostly' together and to take the parent figures as giving us the larger sample.

As can be seen from Table 6.5, the largest proportion (38, 46%) had all or mostly deaf friends, and the vast majority (65, 79%) included some deaf people among their friends. An even greater proportion (73, 89%) included at least some hearing people among their friends. Three-quarters (61/82, 74%) had both deaf and hearing friends. It is not surprising that their preference for deaf or hearing friends showed a significant relationship with their preferred communication.

Most of those who used BSL (23/31) had all or mostly deaf friends, while most of those who were oral (22/30) had all or mostly hearing friends. There was also a relationship with the type of school attended at the secondary stage, as shown in Table 6.6. This is based on parental report and excludes the three attending special units.

Table 6.6. *The relationship between having deaf or hearing friends in adult life and school attended at the secondary stage*

	School for the deaf	PHU	Mainstream
Equal deaf and hearing	8	3	0
All/mostly deaf	28	8	1
All/mostly hearing	5	12	10
No friends	4	0	0

Table 6.7. *Gender differences in friendship patterns*

	Men	Women
Equal deaf and hearing	6	5
All/mostly deaf	15	23
All/mostly hearing	22	6
No friends	5	0

Excluding those with no friends, there is a statistically significant relationship between school attended and friendship pattern ($\chi^2 = 27.234$, $p < 0.001$). Those attending schools for the deaf were much more likely to have all or mostly deaf friends, whereas those who attended mainstream schools were more likely to have all or mostly hearing friends. Clearly this result is not surprising and does not suggest a causal relationship, but that those pupils for whom special education was judged the most suitable were more likely to have deaf friends, while for those for whom mainstream was chosen, hearing friends were more likely.

More interesting is the finding that there were gender differences in friendship patterns, as shown in Table 6.7. All of those with no friends were young men, the majority of these (4/5) being drawn from the group with limited language skills. Young women were significantly more likely to have deaf friends than were young men ($\chi^2 = 13.934$, $p < 0.01$)

PARTNERS

It's best deaf with deaf

Hearing partners are best

For those involved in a stable relationship, this was more often with a deaf then with a hearing person. Of the 82 young people whose parents were

Table 6.8. *Preferred language and partners*

	BSL	SSE	Oral	LLS
Partner	13	7	8	0
No partner	18	6	22	8

interviewed, five were married, a further five were living with a partner, and 18 had a steady girlfriend or boyfriend. Of the remaining 54, 33 (40% of total sample) had never had such a relationship. We did ask the young people about gay and lesbian relationships and one young woman, at her interview, said that she was a lesbian. None of the parents mentioned that their son or daughter was gay or lesbian. As might be expected, the older ones in the sample were more likely to have stable relationships, though, even in this group, the majority did not. Of those over 21 years, a greater proportion (19/48, 40%) had partners compared with those (9/34, 26%) under 21 years. Whether or not they had a partner was not related to preferred language, as is shown in Table 6.8, although none of those with limited language skills had a steady relationship. However, young women were more likely to have partners, or to have had partners (29/34, 85%) than were young men (20/48, 42%).

At the time of the young people interviews, 24 of those interviewed had partners; 19 were deaf and five were hearing. When the young people were asked whether the ideal partner was deaf or hearing, of the 44 who answered, 18 (41%) preferred deaf partners with only six (14%) preferring hearing partners. Of the remainder, 10 (23%) said it depended on the circumstances, and the other 10, (23%) that it did not matter. Of the 19 with deaf partners, 13 favoured deaf partners, but of the five with hearing partners, only one favoured hearing partners.

One of the main reasons for preferring deaf partners was the ease of communication.

It's best deaf with deaf. There's more to talk about when you go out. With hearing people, there's nothing.
Marion, 19 years, BSL

I used to think it would be marvellous to have a hearing boyfriend. I changed my mind when I met my present boyfriend.
Tina, 18 years, oral

Sometimes experience with a hearing boyfriend or girlfriend had led to this conclusion.

My ex-girlfriend was hearing. It wasn't worth it for me. I am lucky now
I have a deaf girlfriend, so there is no problem () it must be a deaf
girlfriend, as they recognise the limitations of the deaf world.
Phillip, 19 years, SSE

Where hearing partners were preferred, pragmatic reasons were often
given, such as the access they could provide to the hearing world.

Hearing partners are best, because I don't know everything; hearing
people know everything.
Tom, 20 years, BSL

It's better with a hearing person; they can help with phone messages. I
wouldn't have to take time off work to sort things out face to face.
Mark, 20 years, oral

I want a hearing woman, not a deaf one. That's not for me. I want a
hearing person, better for emergencies, for the phone and the like.
Sam, 18 years, BSL   .

As with friendships, young women were more likely to have and to prefer a
deaf partner than a hearing one and more likely to emphasise the need for
communication in a relationship. Seventeen of the young women had
partners of whom 16 were deaf and one was hearing, while seven of the
young men had partners of whom three were deaf and four were hearing.
Of the 18 preferring deaf partners, 11 were young women and seven were
young men, and of the six preferring hearing partners, five were young men
and one was a young woman.

Parents generally felt that relationships with deaf partners carried more
promise of success than those with hearing partners, although a number
had not always held this view. The majority of the young people's partners
at the time of the parent interviews were deaf (22/28), with only a minority
being hearing.

I mean, a lot of people think that it is better for them to marry someone
who can hear, because it makes their life better, but they could be
unhappy. There could be frustration, whereas if they marry someone
who's deaf, they are on the same par – on the same level – and they could
possibly be happier. It's just a matter of his happiness. That is what you
want, really.
Mother of Shaun, 21 years, BSL

I think for a time they have to be with people with the same handicap.
That is what I feel personally...Robert is very much for the deaf; now

whether it is different for girls who can mix with hearing boys I don't know, but I can't imagine Robert mixing with a hearing girl, having a hearing girlfriend.
Mother of Robert, 22 years, BSL

The majority of them (boyfriends) are deaf. We wanted deaf, you see, you feel more secure. I don't think a hearing person and a deaf person works. She'd only had hearing people before. I think they took advantage of her
Mother of Teresa, 22 years, BSL

I think they would probably have more in common, you know that they know what the problems are – what problems they have been through – where if you have a hearing person, they can't possibly know how a deaf person thinks or how they feel. So I think a deaf person would be more sympathetic to a deaf person's problems.
Mother of Rosemary, 21 years, oral

The parents who looked for hearing partners for their young people were in a minority, but they also expressed it in terms of wanting their son or daughter to be happy.

In all honesty, yes, (concerning her disappointment that her son has a deaf girlfriend) I was, but my motives were that if he married a hearing girl he would be able to communicate well on a one-to-one relationship and it would have widened his horizons. He would have lived, I felt, a fuller life. Whereas marrying a deaf person, his life would have been much narrower, but then on reflection, as time goes on – you see as a Mum, you still feel at the back of your mind, it sounds crazy doesn't it, that one day the miracle is going to happen, and one day he is going to hear. I know now that he is so much more comfortable in a deaf world and all I want is for him to be happy anyway, I want him to have what makes him happiest.
Mother of Colin, 24 years, BSL

The other concern of parents in thinking about partners was the possibility of deaf grandchildren. All of those who raised this, did so in terms of not wanting deaf grandchildren, except one family who were ambivalent.

I was pleased (about the deaf boyfriend) because there was no history of deafness in the family. I was concerned that if she married a deaf person, her children might be deaf.
Mother of Angela, 19 years, oral

Sometimes I think it would be better if they were deaf, because she could cope. Then I think if they were deaf it would be a shame. Two more deaf, sometimes I'm not sure.
Mother of Shirley, 22 years, SSE

Usually they would arrange the marriage but they don't mind

For some families from the Asian community, there was a particular concern as the parents saw themselves as having a significant involvement in the choice of marriage partner. Some felt, though, the deafness meant that their involvement might be less than with hearing sons and daughters, and only concerned with the endorsement or otherwise of the choice.

I want him married off now, to see if we can find a nice girl. Well, I keep telling him it's time: and he wants to marry a deaf girl.
Interviewer: What do you think?
Well, I want what he wants; the reason is that they can communicate and they can work everything out together. With the hearing girl, he will have so many problems. I would have a problem as well, because it's very difficult to make them understand (his problems). I would rather have a deaf girl. He knows a lot of them; most of his friends are deaf.
Mother of Ritesh, 24 years, BSL

Usually they would arrange the marriage, but they don't mind if he meets someone, as long as it's a nice woman. It will have to be agreed anyway. It could be a deaf or hearing woman as long as they can understand each other.
Sister, interpreting for parents of Kunal, 24 years, BSL

I am looking for a suitable girl. If he wants a girl that can hear and speak it could be difficult. () It's his choice. I've given him the chance. You can have a deaf girl if you want or you can have a hearing girl if you want. We'll try our best to get a hearing girl if that's what you want. If you want a deaf girl and you've got someone in mind you must tell us, and we'll go for it.
Father of Anil, 23 years, BSL

This family was also concerned about the future of any children.

Our main worry is when he gets married as to whether they will live together (meaning together with the parents) or not. That depends on the boy and his partner, that is the main worry. And then the children

they have, that's another problem, because if you don't hear you can't speak and his children could have a problem as well. That is our main worry. That is why we are thinking of a normal girl that can speak and hear.
Father of Anil, 23 years, BSL

LONELINESS

How did you get her to be your friend?

There were very few in the group of young people who were total loners with no social contacts and only one described himself as without friends.

I'm trying to be more sociable. I am trying to eliminate everything unsociable and try and make more friends. I had a penfriend – that collapsed, and that depressed me. I'm easily depressed. I've had no professional help; some people like to go to agony aunts, to trained counsellors. I don't like going on about my emotions. I keep them to myself. I have been a loner all my life...I keep things to myself. It's very hard, I've no-one to talk to, I'm not close to...(sister). I've never felt close to anyone in all my life. I feel tense all the time. I rarely have friends, I never get close.
Francis, 19 years, oral

While this extreme form of loneliness described in the quote above was rare, many more experienced periods of loneliness or feelings of not belonging, as the quote from Christopher at the beginning of this chapter indicates.

Parents, too, commented on the loneliness felt by the young people.

He came back drunk once and I said to him, 'What are you doing getting drunk?' and he said, 'Mum, there were all these teenagers and they were all talking to each other and I had nothing to do so I kept drinking'.
Mother of Andrew, 21 years, BSL

Although he has his own friends he does, in another way, tend to be a loner. He is happier in his own company.
Mother of David, 21 years, oral

Interviewer: And did he talk about being lonely or were you just aware that he was lonely?
I asked him. I discovered the situation. And then he said, 'Yes'. I said, 'Do you cry?' and he said, 'Sometimes'.
Mother of Robert, 22 years, BSL

Yes, I think she is lonely. I think this is why she is always so desperate to have another boyfriend when she loses one. She has got to get someone else and this is what worries us, because they are not always suitable. () She has this desperate need for company. She has never had a close friend at all, never.
Mother of Carol, 23 years, oral

Carol, the young person mentioned above, actually asked her mother about how to make friends.

I mean, I have got a friend I have had since I was 11, and Carol can never quite get over this. She is Carol's god-mother, actually. And she often used to say to me, 'How did you get Aunty Mary?' and 'How did you get her to be your friend?' We were at school together, we sat next to each other, we got on well together, you know. But she has never managed it, has she, to find a friend, not even among the deaf girls.
Mother of Carol, 23 years, oral

Often it was keenly felt in terms of not having a boyfriend or girlfriend as these parents describe. Of the 48 young people over 21 years, 18 (38%) were reported by their parents never to have had a boyfriend or girlfriend.

He has not had a relationship of any description with a girl. () Well, he says to me, 'I'm not bothered' but deep down I can see that he is a bit. He keeps saying, 'I want to buy a house and do this and that' and I say, 'You should wait until you're married'. 'Oh, I'll never get married – what girl would have me?' kind of thing. So he downs himself in that way. I am not sure if it's because he is deaf or because he is Nigel.
Mother of Nigel, 19 years, oral

It is difficult for him to get girlfriends. He's deteriorated since he's got older. He has become more self-conscious. I think he's lonely.
Mother of Gary, 20 years, oral

He's always on about how he can't get a girlfriend and things like that. A lot of them just don't want to know…They don't want to know, they won't talk to him, he's had no steady girlfriends and he's upset.
Mother of Ivan, 21 years, BSL

The young people were less likely to comment on this in such an elaborate way, although Ivan, whose mother is quoted above, did.

I'd be happier if I had a girlfriend. I would go to the pub, play darts and snooker. I want a girlfriend to make my social life better.
Ivan, 21 years, BSL

It was particularly sad if deafness was seen as a barrier to such relationships. Nigel, whose mother is quoted above, felt this.

> *No, I don't think I will get a girlfriend, because I am deaf. I won't get a*
> *girlfriend or get married. I think I would get a girlfriend if I wasn't deaf.*
> *I don't think it will happen in the future.*
> *Interviewer: What do you mean?*
> *I don't feel good enough to be with a girl without hearing, maybe I don't*
> *have the confidence.*
> *Nigel, 19 years, oral*

THE ROLE OF PARENTS

I expect I have taken the place of friends

In some families, parents felt they had a greater role than they would have had had their son or daughter been hearing, in that they themselves were part of their social life and took the place of other friends.

> *Whereas with Joe, from the age of 14, if I wanted to go out, I would have*
> *gone out, but with Bobby, I never wanted to leave him. He was lonely*
> *enough with his deafness, without me going out and leaving him, so I*
> *always tried to be there. () I do worry about the future for him. I'd like*
> *him to go out and meet more people, have a more independent life. I*
> *think if he does not do it now, as he gets older he won't do it. He'll live a*
> *very lonely life.*
> *Mother of Bobby, 20 years, SSE*

> *Friends of her own age, both male and female – I would like her to be in*
> *more contact with them, but there is not a lot to talk about and it is more*
> *interesting to go out with us, or stay at home to watch something on the*
> *television that we can discuss afterwards, () laugh about together. I*
> *expect I have taken the place of friends.*
> *Mother of Helen, 23 years, SSE*

This arrangement was not always satisfactory for either party, and in some cases was a cause of concern for the parents.

> *He'll say he doesn't want a girlfriend. He says he's going to stop with me*
> *at home. The relationship we have now is not healthy. It's too much*
> *with me. I do worry about it these last couple of years. He should be*
> *going out.*
> *Mother of Matthew, 21 years, LLS*

Another way in which parents could be involved in their son's or daughter's life was in assisting in contacting friends and sometimes taking responsibility for quite elaborate arrangements and the parents often had an active role in maintaining the contact between the young people and their friends. As was mentioned in chapters 3 and 5, many of the group were not letter writers, and most could not communicate over the telephone. Moreover, many had friends at a distance, and as has already been shown, many travelled extensively to keep in contact with their friends.

Both parents and young people reported that normally contact was maintained through prearranged meetings. However, the telephone was also a significant means of communication, and in some cases the parents had to mediate or take responsibility for making arrangements.

It's everything you have to do. Paula was going to B. . . last weekend and she didn't know she was going. () Her friend now is married and lives in B. . . so I phoned her mother in L. . . and said 'Paula's going to B. . . to a dance, so it would be nice if she could see Julie'. She said, 'Yes it would be nice, but how can I tell her?' I said, 'I don't know'. So she said, 'I know, I'll phone Peter's father (Julie's husband's father) who lives three miles away and ask him to go and tell them'. So she phones Peter's father, who was in the middle of watching the snooker, which he likes. He left the snooker to drive to Julie's on the chance of them being in, I mean it was not even certain on a Saturday afternoon that they would be in, then drive back. Then they phoned me to tell Paula that 'Yes, they would be in'.
Mother of Paula, 24 years, BSL

FRIENDSHIPS AND RELATIONSHIPS IN EARLY LIFE

The diversity of experience of relationships in our sample was striking, from those with active social lives to others who felt lonely for much of the time. We are able, from our data, to examine whether these later friendships reflect early experience, social competence demonstrated at an earlier stage, or school experience.

Early experiences

Few of the children were at school at the time of the early interviews and attendance at playgroup and nursery school was not as common as it is now. However, the early interviews did contain questions relating to the

Table 6.9. *Early social competence and ability to make friends as a young adult*

	Good skills as child	Poor skills as child
Makes friends easily	11	2
Some difficulty	16	4
Does not make friends easily	14	13

sociability of the child. A scale of social skills was devised, based on whether or not they made themselves understood easily with other children, whether or not they were able to share toys, the extent to which they understood about taking it in turns and their understanding of games that had a winner. Good skills were classified as a positive response to three or four of the questions, whereas poor skills were indicated by a two or fewer positive responses. Table 6.9 shows the relationship between early social competence and the ability as young people to make friends. The table is based on the 60 of the sample who were three and a half years or over at the first interview, and parental report of later friendship patterns.

Thus, the majority of those who make friends easily as young adults had good skills as a child, although those who do not make friends easily now varied in their skills as a child. This is statistically significant, ($\chi^2 = 6.240$, $p < 0.05$). However, the amount that the young people played with other children as a child, whether or not their parents felt they were left out of games when young, and whether or not they were submissive or bossy with other children, did not show statistical relationships with patterns of friendships as an adult, as reported by the parents or by the young people themselves.

School experiences

When she was at boarding school, she was lonely

I made lots of friends. I remember lots of happy times

School is an important consideration, because of the important role of school friendships in early adult life, as has already been mentioned, but also because the debate around appropriate education for deaf children places emphasis on the school experience. As was pointed out earlier, a direct relationship between type of school attended and the maintenance of school friendships into adult life was not sustained. All forms of schooling included some children who kept their friends into adulthood and some who did not.

Both parents and young people were asked about friendship patterns at secondary school and a similar pattern emerged to that in their reports of current friendships. The majority had stable friendships, either a special friend or a group of stable friends, but again the parents saw less stability in the relationships than did the young people. Overall in the interviews, the parents were more likely in the comments they made to emphasise the difficulties their sons and daughters had in relationships, while the young people overall were much more positive in their accounts.

Almost a third (25/82) of the deaf children in the study were described by their parents as having difficulties making friends at school. Parents tended in their interviews to stress these difficulties.

> *I used to think of him as a bit of a loner at school. I have never known him have a best friend, no.*
> *Mother of Mark, 22 years, oral*

> *Interviewer: Was he ever lonely?*
> *Yes, I think so. He seemed to live in his own little world.*
> *Mother of Bobby, 20 years, SSE*

> *When she was at boarding school she was lonely. She found it hard to make friendships, particularly with girls.*
> *Mother of Tina, 18 years, oral*

One of the problems perceived by parents was the distance between home and school, which made the maintenance of friendships difficult. Friendships were formed with other deaf children at school, but because of the distance separating the children's homes, there were few opportunities for mutual visits out of school hours.

> *Interviewer: Did he make any friends at L...?*
> *Oh yes, one or two.*
> *Interviewer: Did he bring any home or not?*
> *No, they didn't come, because it was too far.*
> *Mother of Edward, 23 years, oral*

> *You see, the thing is, when they are away from home and they are not going to a local school, they have no local friends. Really, they are isolated, aren't they? You make your friends at school, don't you, and if you are not at the local school, you haven't got any local friends.*
> *Mother of Trevor, 22 years, oral*

A second issue could be communication difficulties experienced by the children, making interaction difficult, as this parent describes:

> *Interviewer: When she was a little girl did she like to play on her own, or did she like to play with other children?*
> *Play on her own.*
> *Interviewer: Is that all the time?*
> *Yes, because they wouldn't have anything to do with her, because they couldn't understand her and she couldn't understand them.*
> *Interviewer: Was she ever lonely?*
> *Probably, yes.*
> *Mother of Mary, BSL, 23 years*

Other parents described to us how friendships made could be different.

> *They make friends at school but they tend to be the odd children. On the whole you find that they are not mixing. They are the 'hardwork kids', they don't make friends easily.*
> *Mother of Fiona, 22 years, SSE*

> *He likes to move round with his friends. He had a particular friend at P... He always goes for the underdog.*
> *Mother of Gary, 20 years, oral*

> *The same thing happens at work as happened at school. () Always seems to be somebody with a disadvantage herself that is a bit more friendly to Carol. I don't mean they are nasty to her. I make sure they are not. I think, on the whole, they are very friendly with a deaf girl and there aren't that many people that are willing to take that trouble. It is in a way sad, very sad really, but it always seems to be as I say, somebody with a disadvantage of some kind who will take the trouble to be a bit more friendly to Carol.*
> *Mother of Carol, 23 years, oral*

However, many of the young people enjoyed their time at school, because of the friends they had there. When asked what they liked most about school, of the 51 who could answer, 45 (88%) gave responses referring to some aspect of the social side. For nearly one-third (16, 31%) of them it was the only thing they identified. Isabel, whose story starts this book, said:

> *I liked W..., as there were many people, lots of different subjects. It was very strict but that did not bother me, as we were all very close.*
> *Isabel, 21 years, SSE*

Janet, too, talked of closeness at school.

> *Good times with my school friends? Oh, I had better not say this, but we used to do a lot of things together. I was especially close to the boys; we used to go around like brothers and sisters; it was lovely. We used to do lots of things together, trusted each other, it was really good. I think some of the things we wouldn't have done if we'd not been so close.*
> *Janet, 22 years, oral*

Tina's parent described her as lonely at boarding school (see above) yet she herself said:

> *I was there for seven years. I made lots of friends. I remember lots and lots of happy times.*
> *Tina, 18 years, oral*

INFLUENCES ON SOCIAL LIFE

A number of factors emerged in the discussion of friendship patterns. The preferred language of the young people showed no relationship with how well they made friends, except that those with very limited skills all had great difficulty. Not surprisingly, preferred language and type of school attended showed a relationship with the preference for deaf or hearing friends. Those whose preferred language was BSL and those who attended special schools for the deaf were significantly more likely to have deaf friends. The degree of hearing loss did not make a difference to ease of making friends. Of the sample, 20% (16/82) were said by their parents to make friends easily. These were spread across the range of hearing losses (profoundly deaf, 5/31, 16%; severely deaf, 6/30, 20%; and moderately deaf or partially hearing, 5/21, 23%).

Interestingly, there was a relationship between some aspects of early social competence and later friendship patterns. In addition, however, it was shown that women were more likely than men to prefer deaf friends. This may be because of the different social activities of men and women, or because women put a higher emphasis on compatible communication within their relationships.

Overall, an extremely complex pattern of social relationships emerged from the research. Firstly, there was a wide range of social experience, from very active social lives to feelings of isolation and loneliness. Secondly, the perceptions of the young people and their parents differed in some respects. The majority of parents did not feel their son or daughter really enjoyed the kind of social life which they felt was the norm.

Some parents regretted the absence of an imagined ease they felt should exist in the formation of friendships at this stage in their children's lives.

> *I don't know what it's like for Jean to come in and say, 'I haven't got time for dinner, Mum, I'm going out', and bringing different girlfriends home.*
> Mother of Jean, 22 years, SSE

> *Brenda she is quite friendly with, but she never sees her other than at the Deaf Club. This is the sort of thing I never quite understand about these...whether they invite other people to their houses or what, I don't know, but they never invited Carol to their home ever.*
> Mother of Carol, 23 years, oral

Parents sometimes saw the friendships as very vulnerable.

> *Sometimes I say to her, 'You are being a silly girl here, you know', (about travelling around to meet friends). Then I get this, 'You don't know what it is like to be deaf. It's a small world and you can't afford to lose friends; you have got to keep your friends'. This is what I get, you see.*
> Mother of Isabel, 21 years, SSE

> *She is always scared of losing friends, particularly the deaf friends, not so much hearing people. She seems to me to be a little bit scared of losing deaf friends, because she always says the deaf world is so small!*
> Parent of Janet, 22 years, oral

Most of the young people, however, felt generally happy and described their social life as rich and varied. The reason for the discrepancy between young people's and parent views is interesting. In our opinion it relates to different expectations of friendship in the two groups. However, it could be because of different perceptions by young people and their parents of the situation, or that the two groups elected to focus on different aspects in the interview.

CHAPTER SEVEN

Being deaf

I want people to understand me the way I am – deaf
Mark, 20 years, oral

This chapter is concerned with the way in which the young deaf people saw themselves, and is largely based on information from the interviews with them themselves. Some comparisons with information from their parents are made in the next chapter. It begins by opening the discussion on whether there is such a thing as a typical deaf person. It examines what the young people felt about their own deafness, what it was like to grow up as a deaf person, and the extent to which the young people were involved with the Deaf community and with Deaf politics.

In writing this, we are aware that the young people we interviewed, their families and probably readers of this book will differ in their understanding of what is desirable for deaf people making the transition into adulthood. Some will look to the group to see the extent to which they are proud of being deaf and identify with the Deaf community. Others will see success in terms of the extent to which the young people have been able to minimise the consequences of their deafness, have overcome it and lived their lives alongside hearing people. Within the group, the variety of potentially desirable outcomes arises partly because of the diversity of the group, based as it is on those parents and children recruited at the preschool stage, because the children were known to have a hearing loss. Other recent studies, with samples that were selected at the time the research was carried out, have focused on more specific groups, such as those who attended schools for the deaf (Denmark *et al.*, 1979), those who were profoundly deaf (Kyle & Allsop, 1982), those who were members of Deaf Clubs (Jackson, 1986), those who were integrated at school (Lynas,

1986), those known to Social Services (Sainsbury, 1986), or those known to services for hearing impaired children (Moore & Beazley, 1991). For these groups, the likelihood of identification with the Deaf community or the hearing world was more clearly specified at the outset.

In this chapter, we start by looking, in general, at personality characteristics and attitudes to being deaf. We then examine the extent to which the young people felt themselves to be members of the Deaf community and their political awareness. Later in the chapter we look at specific, but disparate, groups within the sample that seem to warrant attention, including those who identified exclusively with the hearing world, those from minority ethnic communities, those whose language skills limited their participation in the research and those about whom we ourselves felt concern. We conclude by considering the extent to which the young people felt their deafness affected their parents' lives.

A DEAF PERSONALITY?

Much of the literature on deafness has tended to endorse the idea that there is a specific deaf personality which is generally described in negative terms. Rodda & Grove (1987), reviewing this literature, suggested that deaf people 'are said to exhibit a lack of sensitivity to others, over dependence, unsociability, impatience and to react to frustration with anger and overt aggression'. In this chapter and the next, we consider, by looking at the young people's accounts and their parents' views, whether it is possible to attribute specific characteristics to deaf people.

During the interview, we asked the young people what kind of person they felt themselves to be. We prompted them on whether they felt themselves to be generally happy or sad, calm or easily worked up, creative with lots of ideas, confident or not confident, whether or not they could trust people, and whether or not they were the sort of person who could show their feelings easily or who kept themselves to themselves. Some found the question easy to answer and gave a description with very little prompting.

> *(giggles) I love eating, but I am going on a sponsored slim. I am very shy, but I like going out. I love staying in the bath a long time. I'm very untidy. I'm a terrible person. I like being quiet, but I have lots of hobbies: knitting, sewing, patchwork.*
> *Carol, 23 years, oral*

It was clear, though, that many of the young people found it difficult to

Table 7.1. *Young people's view of aspects of their own personality*

	Yes		Varies		No		
	Number	%	Number	%	Number	%	Not answered
Happy	35	65	13	24	6	11	7
Calm	18	39	14	30	14	30	15
Confident	19	40	20	42	9	19	13
Shows feelings	13	29	20	44	12	27	16

answer such questions, even when prompted. Often, they had never thought of themselves in this way before, and had very rarely been asked to describe themselves. A summary of the results for some of these characteristics is given in Table 7.1.

It was encouraging to see that most of the young people, nearly two-thirds, described themselves as happy and only one in ten as not happy. In terms of calmness, just over one-third who answered saw themselves as calm, while just under one-third felt they became 'easily worked up'. While four out of ten felt generally confident, for a further four out of ten, whether or not they felt confident depended upon the situation, and one in five never felt confident. Likewise, for more than four out of ten whether or not they showed their feelings depended on the situation, although about one quarter felt they were never able to show how they felt.

As might be expected, the question on how easy or not it was to trust other people gave rise to complex replies and we have not attempted to quantify the answers, which covered a range of possible responses.

I have too much trust in other people. If they let me down I lose heart.
Ruth, 19 years, oral

I hold back at first, if I don't know people very well, but later on I will tell secrets or confidential things.
Josie, 24 years, BSL

I don't find it easy to trust people. I know I can trust some people, but not many. I show my feelings to my family, but not to outsiders.
Tina, 18 years, oral

We also asked the young people whether they had any particular anxieties. All except for one could answer this question and the majority (36/60, 60%) could think of nothing in particular about which they were anxious.

We then went on to probe in depth how the young people felt about themselves as people, and asked questions related to their self esteem.

Table 7.2. *The self esteem of the deaf young people*

	Yes		Varies		No		
	Number	%	Number	%	Number	%	Not answered
Likes self	37	70	10	19	6	11	8
Proud of self	26	55	13	28	8	17	14
Sorry for self	24	42	16	28	17	30	4
Wants to change self	34	64	4	8	15	28	8

Do you like yourself?

Do you ever feel proud of yourself?

Do you ever feel sorry for yourself?

Is there anything about yourself you do not like and want to change?

Although these are difficult and personal questions, most of the young people were very frank in their responses. A summary of their replies is given in Table 7.2. Although one in ten did not like themselves and one in six never felt proud of themselves, the majority liked themselves and sometimes felt proud of themselves.

I felt proud of myself, because I thought I would never get a job and I've got one.
Richard, 20 years, oral

Of the 24 who felt sorry for themselves, in seven instances, this was related to specific events rather than feeling sorry for themselves in a general way. Because of the way in which they understood the question, of the 34 who wanted to change themselves, nearly one third (11) referred to specific concrete changes they would like to make, usually to physical aspects of themselves. Nearly half of those answering this question (23/53, 43%) wanted to make changes to some aspect of their personality.

I would like to have more patience; I don't suffer fools gladly.
Jane, 20 years, oral

Sometimes I don't like myself when I lose my temper.
Tina, 18 years, oral

A picture emerges of a group of young people, of whom the majority liked themselves and felt proud of themselves, although most of them had aspects of themselves they would have liked to change. The most negative finding was that the majority did feel sorry for themselves. No consistent personality patterns appeared to emerge, and a range of personality characteristics was described, as it might with any group of young people. There was nothing in the responses of the young people to suggest a specific Deaf personality and the notion of a 'Deaf psychology' is discussed further in the next chapter.

BEING DEAF

I am happy as I am, deaf

I hoped I would be hearing. () When I was young – that was the bad time, I remember the pain

We also asked the young people a series of questions about being deaf, which it was hoped would tap their feelings about it. These were nearly the last questions in the schedule, and so were asked after some considerable time reflecting on deafness. We were particularly interested to see whether they would reflect the view generally held by society that sees deafness as an impairment and thus negative, or whether some of them would have developed a positive Deaf identity and perhaps saw themselves as a member of a thriving Deaf community.

One way in which we examined this was to ask about the extent to which they felt their life might have been different had they been hearing. This is a controversial question, because of the possible implication that to be hearing is somehow better (see Appendix III). The implication that deaf people are different was one that was rejected by eight of the group.

All my life I have been saying I am no different to anyone.
Michael, 20 years, oral

Only three of the sample felt that they themselves would not be different, seeing aspects of their basic personality over-riding any effect of deafness.

No. I would be the same as I am now. Moaning and getting into trouble.
Harry, 20 years, BSL

However, the vast majority (46/57, 81%) of those able to answer this question described areas of difference and of these nearly half (21/46, 46%) specified a number of ways in which their lives would be different. The others concentrated on one specific aspect, nearly one third (14/46, 30%) focused on relationships, six (13%) on differences in the area of work, and five (11%) on differences relating to hearing or speaking. However, this does not give a complete picture, as the differences specified were not necessarily exclusively positive or negative. In the area of friendships and relationships, which was a major concern, some, for example, felt their social life was restricted by their deafness.

I think there would be some advantages (in being hearing). I could make more friends at work, make more conversations, be able to make jokes.
Carol, 23 years, oral

I'd be more open like all hearing people. I'd have more friends, it would be easier to make friends, everything would be easier.
Nicky, 21 years, SSE

But there were others who saw their lives as enriched in that they had more friends.

I think I would be here (university). I would read at the same level, but I wouldn't be as happy. I am happy, because I know I have got friends everywhere. Hearing people don't have the same sort of contact. I wouldn't get so much out of life.
Ray, 21 years, oral

If I was hearing I would have friends only from my local home area, but being deaf I have friends all over the place. I think that deaf social life is better than hearing social life. The hearing people at work think that deaf people have a better social life.
Rosemary, 21 years, oral

Yes, because I am regularly in the deaf world; weekends and so on I spend with deaf friends. Only Thursday night do I go for a drink with hearing people. If I was hearing, life would not be as good. There'd be discos but sport would be worse. Deaf people have a lot of sport.
Paula, 24 years, BSL

This, of course, reinforces the comments made by some of the young people about their social life in the previous chapter.

Those deaf people who focused on work as an area of difference, however, were more likely to see negative consequences of their deafness. A common response referred to their inability to join the forces. Some reached their conclusions by drawing comparisons with their siblings or contemporaries. For others, their aspirations had not been realised and they attributed this (rightly or wrongly) to their deafness.

It would not make any difference apart from being able to join the army.
Geoffrey, 21 years, oral

I think I would have followed in my sister's footsteps; she did what a hearing person does: she went to a hearing school, she went on to university, got herself a good job afterwards. She is on a good salary and I think if I had good hearing I would have gone on and got good A-levels and gone to university. I think that is the way I would have gone, but because I am deaf, it held me back a bit, but I don't regret it at all.
Janet, 22 years, oral

Yes, life would be different. I would be a famous sportsman.
Richard, 20 years, oral

I would hear everything, talk, use the phone, maybe challenge in politics – it would be a big change.
Isabel, 21 years, SSE

I don't mind being deaf but if I was hearing I could have got a job modelling.
Shirley, 22 years, SSE

Only one saw his deafness as contributing positively to his career.

I would be on the dole, because I would not be so determined, or I would have got a nine-to-five job, as I would not be so motivated. Probably I would have joined the forces (he now works at a sports centre).
Jeremy, 20 years, oral

Some answered the question by talking about their own personal development, many of them stressing that deafness had become an integral part of their identity and personality.

It could be different. I don't know. Most of the time I'm glad I'm deaf.
Brenda, 21 years, SSE

I don't think I would be as sensitive as I am now. I would be a different character altogether. I certainly would not be as understanding, because I know what it is like for people to have to try and understand me, so I probably would not have been so patient either. If I had my hearing now I don't think I would cope, though obviously I would have to. I am coping all right now, I am quite happy the way I am. I don't know, it's a difficult question.
Ruth, 19 years, oral

Table 7.3. *Times when the young people*
wished they were hearing

	Number	%
In past only	27	49
Past and now	22	40
Now only	4	7
Never	2	3

Seeing deafness as an intrinsic aspect of themselves also emerged in answers to a question about whether they had ever wished they were hearing. The results are given in Table 7.3, for the 55 who answered the question. Of these, 53 (97%) had at some time wished to be hearing and only 2 (3%) had never wished to be hearing. However, for nearly half of them the wish to be hearing was one they had held in the past but not now. Just over half of them, at the time of the interview, did not wish they were hearing and just under half wished they were.

When I found out, I was upset and cried. I wished I could be hearing. I was about ten years old. Now I'm not bothered.
Marion, 19 years, BSL

I used to argue with my mother when I was seven or eight years old, 'Why am I deaf and my brothers hearing?' Now I'm not bothered, I enjoy myself, I have deaf friends.
Christopher, 21 years, BSL

I wanted to be hearing when I was small, because people laughed at me. Now I am not bothered.
Ivan, 21 years, BSL

When I was ten, I asked Mum to change me from being deaf to being hearing to send me to hospital. Mum explained that all deaf people would like to be like that, to change to hearing. She explained hearing people and deaf people are different; hearing people have 'open ears' and deaf people have 'closed ears'.
Gary, 20 years, oral

When I was young I asked the teacher, 'Is it possible to become hearing?' I hoped I would become hearing.
Interviewer: What about your friends?
They were the same. We talked about it; we all wanted to become hearing. I hoped I would become hearing.

Interviewer: So there was a time when you wished you were hearing?
When I was young – that was the bad time, I remember the pain.
Interviewer: Do you now? Not now.
Phillip, 19 years, SSE

For some the reasons for wanting to be hearing were, or had been, practical.

Quite a lot of times, especially at critical times such as when there is no monitor board at railway stations.
Francis, 19 years, oral

There was a time when the Stereo Walkman came in I wished I was hearing, so I could see what they were like.
Interviewer: Now?
No.
Paula, 24 years, BSL

Yes of course. When I want information on something on TV and there is no teletext. When I'm in a group of hearing people. Not really now.
Ray, 21 years, oral

For others it was related to the desire to communicate more easily.

Yes, a few times, so I could make friends locally with people who live across the road, it would be easier to talk to people like hairdressers and teachers. My mother is a teacher and sometimes I would like to be a teacher like her.
Interviewer: Do you now?
No, I don't wish I was hearing.
Brenda, 21 years, SSE

When I'm down the pub. My dad wears a hearing aid and he finds it difficult in the pub as well.
Malcolm, 22 years, oral

When I was nine I had friends who were hearing and I was always the last to know what was going on, such as jokes. I felt left out.
Interviewer: Do you now?
No.
Rosemary, 21 years, oral

Yes, I wanted to be hearing and learn to speak. I was fed up with signing. Now I am not bothered.
Bridget, 22 years, BSL

Many explained how deafness was an integral part of their personality now they were older.

> *Not really now, because if I became hearing it would mean lots of changes.*
> *Tina, 18 years, oral*

> *If I was hearing I don't know how I would cope with it. It would be like a completely different way of life.*
> *Ruth, 19 years, oral*

> *No, if there was an operation to become hearing I would not have it.*
> *Deborah, 20 years, oral*

> *Maybe when I was younger, but not now. I was born for it.*
> *Zoe, 19 years, BSL*

> *No, I am happy as I am, deaf. Its too late for me to become hearing now. I used to want to hear before, so I would be able to talk to people and understand them.*
> *Harry, 20 years, BSL*

> *Never. I can't change into a hearing person now – it's too late. I don't worry about it.*
> *Amy, 19 years, BSL*

When I was little I believed that one day I would hear

What is interesting about this is not only that they were more likely to have wished to be hearing in the past than now, but that some had felt it was a possibility. Deaf people have for a long time told stories of how they had believed as children that when they became adults they would become hearing. Presumably this arose because many deaf children never saw deaf adults. It is hardly surprising for children in those schools for the deaf where all the children were deaf and all the adults hearing. This research gave us the opportunity to ask specifically about this and one-third (19/57, 33%) reported that they had at some time thought they would become hearing when they grew up.

> *I was nine or ten when I first went to Deaf Club. That was the first time I realised that adults could be deaf and not just children. When I was young I thought everybody was deaf, but as I grew older I realised it was not everybody, but then I thought it was only children. Then when I saw*

deaf adults, I realised that they could be deaf too – and I realised I would grow up to be a deaf adult.
Helen, 23 years, SSE

When I was in the second year at H…, I'd never met a deaf adult, so I told Mum, 'When I grow up I will be hearing like all the teachers are hearing'. I was upset when she told me I would always be deaf. I was worried I would be the only one, that there would be no other deaf adults.
Ray, 21 years, oral

I thought that once, when I was very young, four or five. I thought my hearing would improve. I didn't realise I was deaf. By seven or eight I realised I would be deaf permanently.
Isabel, 21 years, SSE

I felt angry when I first knew I was deaf. When I was 18 I tried to find out whose fault it was. Mark, my friend, said it was my fault. At 14 I thought I would be hearing, but Mum explained to me that I would always be deaf.
Edward, 23 years, oral

For others becoming hearing was not related to being adult but just something that would happen.

I imagined one day there would be a pop in my ears and I would become hearing.
Gary, 20 years, oral

While in the early years, deaf children may not have had a clear idea about their own deafness, most of them (42, 69%) seem to have realised it by the age of eleven. This was further revealed in a question that concerned the age when they first became aware that they were deaf and not hearing. When asked when they first realised they were deaf, 14 (23%) said they had always known or realised prior to going to school, 28 (46%) said they had realised at the infant junior stage between five and eleven years of age, and only four (7%) at secondary age or over. For 2 (3%) the realisation had come gradually over a long period. Thirteen (21%) did not know when they had realised or could not answer the question. As with the question about how life would be different, a few rejected the question, because they did not feel they were 'different' in the sense of being deaf rather than hearing, and these are included in the last group.

I don't remember, I'm not different.
Daniel, 21 years, oral

I don't regard myself as different. I see what you mean, but I have never thought of it like that even at secondary school. I was always aware of things but did not realise the problems it caused. But I don't regard myself as different.
Ruth, 19 years, oral

Most, however, accepted the question. Some first realised they were not hearing because of other people's response to them.

When I was about a year old. My mother would shout at me, but talk to my brother and he would turn round.
Christopher, 21 years, BSL

I can't remember. Seven or eight, I think. Mum told me to go and buy some flowers. The lady could not understand me. I was upset. I realised, when she gave me paper and pen, I realised I was different from the others.
Ray, 21 years, oral

Because once when we were playing in the playground and I think I was chasing after the boys or something and one of the boys got hold of me and the other boys said, 'Be careful, be careful'. That hit home – they didn't treat the others like they did me.
Janet, 22 years, oral

At school, I saw I was different – they were all talking normally and I realised I was different – the teacher was talking simply to me, differently from the way she talked to other children.
Phillip, 19 years, SSE

But for most of those who realised at the younger ages, it was often the hearing aid that was the clue, being an observable physical entity that made them different from other children. This seemed more important than any notion that they were different in terms of their response to the environment.

When I was very young, about five or six.
Interviewer: What made you aware?
My hearing aids. I thought the whole world had them until then. I took them out but could not hear sounds, so I put them back in and I could hear sounds.
Mark, 20 years, oral

When I was about three or four. I realised it over a few weeks, because I wore hearing aids and others did not.
Jean, 20 years, SSE

I always thought I was different, but I did not know why until I was five or six. I had a body worn aid, and I realised that others did not have them.
Jeremy, 20 years, oral

I was in the class, I was about seven or eight and there was a teacher called Miss... () She took me and Paul, we were in Class 4, just him and me to a normal school just for one afternoon. There was not writing and that, just painting and drawing, like play school. That's when I realised I was different to them because nobody wore hearing aids, they were all talking and they had more fun () and I realised they weren't wearing a hearing aid or signing.
Trevor, 22 years, oral

Some were told they were 'deaf', but the idea did not make any sense to them.

I remember being told, 'You don't hear things, you're deaf' and I thought my brother and sister were deaf, I thought they couldn't hear either. And they said, 'No they can hear'. And I said, 'What does it mean?' as I really did not know what it meant. I did not think that deafness means you don't hear, but it was just a word for me. I didn't know what it meant.
Josie, 24 years, BSL

Others had vivid memories but it could be difficult to interpret them.

When I was about three, I just knew I could not hear. I have a photo and I remember that moment. I remember my brother picking me up on the swing – I couldn't hear him coming and then I saw his face. I remember that vividly.
Zoe, 19 years, BSL

When I was about three or four. Where we used to live there was a deaf pig and one day I went to pick it up and it bit me. That's when I first knew I was deaf.
Geoffrey, 21 years, oral

Geoffrey's story may not be clear from the quote, but from other information it appears that Geoffrey, who was used to pigs, approached this one from behind and took it by surprise. His mother, by way of explanation for the fact that the pig had bitten him, told him that the pig had not known he was there, because it was deaf. At that point Geoffrey remembers realising that he was the same as the pig, that he did not always hear people approaching him from behind.

The situations described here echo those discussed by Padden and Humphries (1988). To sense that one is different from other people is complex. The visible evidence, such as hearing aids are one way, and those young people who described realisation in terms of these generally realised at an earlier age. To feel that one is different in terms of the way one responds to the world is more difficult. Padden and Humphries, in discussing this for hearing children of deaf parents, suggest there is certain evidence. The deaf child may observe that there is always someone there when the parents open the front door, for example. However, a child could easily attribute this to the perceived greater knowledge of adults. In fact in our sample, the understanding often came through comparison with other hearing children rather than adults. Padden and Humphries, in describing the experience of deaf children of deaf parents, suggest that here there may be even less evidence and that realisation may not occur until the child observes other hearing children at school. They describe this as 'learning to be deaf'.

My thoughts are doing the talking

We tried to explore whether the young people ever thought of themselves as hearing by asking whether they were deaf or hearing in their dreams. This is, of course, a difficult question and ten were unable to answer it. Of those who could answer, the largest group thought they were hearing 20 (39%) and for a further 12 (24%) it varied, and only ten (20%) were deaf. A further nine (18%) understood the question but could not say whether they were deaf or hearing.

> *Hearing, because I can talk to everyone.*
> *Mark, 20 years, oral*

> *Hearing, I think. I feel like a normal person.*
> *Francis, 19 years, oral*

> *Both – sometimes I sign and sometimes I talk.*
> *Christopher, 21 years, BSL*

> *I'm hearing. I'm talking like a hearing person.*
> *Carol, 23 years, oral*

I think I talk to hearing people in my dreams.
Diane, 20 years, BSL

I'm hearing. Its difficult to remember – my thoughts are doing the talking.
Keith, 19 years, BSL

Deaf and oral.
Interviewer: How do you know?
Because if I come across a hearing person in a dream, I always say, 'Sorry' or 'Can you write that down please?'
Ray, 21 years, oral

I talk – it's impossible to sign.
Shaun, 21 years, BSL

I'm deaf, but I don't use sign language, I talk.
Zoe, 19 years, BSL

Some commented on how strange it was that they were hearing in their dreams.

I had a funny dream. I was hearing. In another dream I was deaf. When I'm asleep I can hear voices in my ears – I think I'm hearing, but how can I be? I'm not.
Amanda, 20 years, SSE

I sometimes dream I am hearing and talking. Then when I wake up, I am deaf. I can't believe that I can be talking in my dreams.
Amy, 19 years, BSL

Interestingly, those who, at the time of the interview, wished to be hearing were significantly more likely to be always or sometimes hearing in their dreams. ($\chi^2 = 4.126$, $p < 0.05$)

I used to watch to see what my signing looked like in the mirror

Around this whole area of how the young people saw themselves, another interesting point emerged in the interviews, in the discussion of dreams, or imaginary friends or language. This was whether or not they ever watched themselves communicating in the mirror. Because we did not have a direct question about this and it was an issue that emerged spontaneously in some of the interviews, we do not know the actual number that did this, but 12 of them mentioned it, which suggests the number is probably higher than the

20% that this represents. Of these 12, six were BSL users, four SSE users,
and two were oral.

Clearly the function this served for many of the sign users (BSL or SSE)
was to see what their signing looked like, or to build their confidence.

*I communicated with myself and I would watch my hands moving. () I
can't see my own hands that way and I wanted to see what it looked like
to deaf people; that's why I used to do it in the mirror.*
Josie, 24 years, BSL

I used to sign in the mirror. I was trying to make myself more confident.
Christine, 21 years, SSE

*When I was little I made faces in the mirror, played signing to myself,
tried signing in front of the mirror.*
Helen, 23 years, SSE

For the two who were oral it also seemed to serve a function of monitoring
their own appearance when they communicated, although they were the
only two oral young people who mentioned it.

I look at myself in the mirror to see what I look like when I talk.
Ray, 21 years, oral

*I used to talk to myself in the mirror, change faces in the mirror, learn to
be angry in the mirror.*
Mark, 20 years, oral

There was a feeling among this group that this behaviour was odd or
somehow unacceptable.

*I feel embarrassed to tell you this, but I used to put a chair in front of the
mirror and sign to myself. My Mum used to give me strange looks. I
used to watch to see what my signing looked like in the mirror.*
Sam, 18 years, BSL

*I would sign to myself in the mirror. People could see me signing but
there was no-one there. My deaf friends would understand. They said
they used to do the same. My mother caught me in the bathroom one
day signing to myself in the mirror – she was worried and told my Dad.*
Darren, 22 years, BSL

We feel we should end this discussion of what the young people felt about
being deaf, on a cautionary note. In a discussion such as this with a focus
on deafness, there is a danger of attributing everything to this, and thus

Table 7.4. *Attendance at Deaf Club*

	Number	%
Yes	43	77
In the past but not now	3	5
Never	10	18
Could not answer	5	

Table 7.5. *Deaf Club attendance and preferred language*

	BSL	SSE	Oral
Attended	20	11	12
Did not attend	2	0	11

preventing ourselves appropriately considering these as young people in their transition into adulthood. As one said during the group discussion:

I've the right to fail. Because if I fail people say it's because I am deaf but hearing people are allowed to fail, and they can make their excuse. Everybody makes the excuse for my failure my deafness.

Tina, 18 years, oral

THE DEAF COMMUNITY AND DEAF POLITICS

What does disabled mean?

In Chapter 1, we described how for many deaf people the Deaf community is important in their lives and being Deaf is an integral part of their identity. We were interested to find out the extent to which this was the case for these young deaf people. We considered whether they felt themselves to be part of a Deaf community and whether they were concerned with political issues as they affect deaf people. To look at this further, we asked the young people whether they had attended a Deaf Club (see Table 7.4). Deaf Club attendance was, not surprisingly, related to preferred language (see Table 7.5). The differences here were statistically significant ($\chi^2 = 13.603$ $p < 0.01$) Not surprisingly, BSL users were more likely to attend, although half of those whose preferred communication was oral also went.

The parents were asked about Deaf Club membership and it is interesting that the parents gave much lower figures for this. Of the whole

Table 7.6. *Parents' and young people's reports of Deaf Club*

	Parents' report		
	Member	Member in past, not now	Not member
Young person's report			
Attends	29	8	6
Attended in past, not now	1	2	0
Never attended	0	0	10
Could not answer	2	0	3

sample, they suggested that 39 (48%) were members, 14 (17%) were members in the past but not at the time of the interview, and 29 (35%) had never even visited a Deaf Club. If we consider the parents' information only for those for whom we also have information from the young deaf people, there is a discrepancy, as we see in Table 7.6. Whether this discrepancey is due to the disctinction we, inadvertantly, introduced between being a member of a Deaf Club and attending a Deaf Club, we cannot be sure. However, we feel the fact that more young people described visiting a Deaf Club, when their parents said they did not, or were no longer members, may be because parents did not want to see their son or daughter associated with a Deaf Club.

Even if the young people attended Deaf Club, most of them seem to be little involved in the political activity of the Deaf community, or to be informed of the issues that concern the Deaf community: seeking recognition of sign language, stressing the need for more sign language interpreters and requesting more sign language or more subtitles on television. Based on the interviewers' assessment, only eight (13%) seemed involved in these issues, although nearly two-thirds (39, 64%) had some minimal awareness. Nearly one-quarter (14, 23%) had no knowledge of these issues at all. Only seven belonged to any of the major national Deaf organisations, although a further three had been members in the past.

In the group discussions, which were with selected deaf young people, who were chosen because of their willingness to get together and talk about deafness and may not have been representative, we tried to discuss further awareness of Deaf issues. One of these concerned Government provision for deaf people and general awareness of what would be required to give deaf people equal access to work, social life, etc. The discussion ranged from the provision of subtitles and text telephones to equality in employment.

*Janet: Yes, I think they should put more money for access to infor-
mation – it's not difficult to do. All programmes should be subtitled –*

they can't deny that.

Janet: I think there should be Minicoms (text telephones) in all public areas like hospitals and stations.

Tina: See Hear (a BBC programme for deaf and hard-of-hearing people) had an item about public telephones with Minicoms. It's really good in the USA; I hope it will happen in England.

Tina: I'd like more equality in employment. I applied but I didn't say I was deaf, so they didn't know until I got to the interview.

Janet: When I apply for a job I put I'm deaf – I'm not ashamed. I don't know whether it is a good idea or not.

Amanda: I found out that a deaf lorry driver has been banned. The Government don't believe that deaf people can drive lorries.

Andrew: I know why. It's because they can't hear what's going on. Like if they've run over someone and they're screaming.

Tina: Well if you think about it, it's the same for a hearing person.

Kerry: And hearing people drive with the radio on.

Andrew: Well, with a lorry it's hard to see out of the back window.

Overall, the young deaf people seemed to feel that necessary equipment was not always provided and that deaf people could be victims of discrimination. The group then addressed the more controversial issue as to whether deaf people are disabled or whether they should be considered as a linguistic and cultural minority group. Many deaf people now consider there are sufficient grounds to demand recognition of Deaf people as a minority group: their language, their history, their art forms and their way of life. For some, this means they should no longer be considered as disabled. The young people were asked about the extent to which they saw themselves as disabled.

Interviewer: What do you think about being registered disabled? Do you think it is positive?

Jeremy: How many here are registered disabled?

(A show of hands indicated all except Jeremy).

Jeremy: I was asked to sign it by a top councillor, because it would be good for the image of the council. I told them what they could do with the paper. I see it as an insult to those who are profoundly deaf or in wheelchairs or worse off than me. I wouldn't sign the paper.

Interviewer: It's an insult to whom?

Jeremy: To people who are worse off than me.

Interviewer: But is it an insult to you?

Jeremy: Yes, because I don't see it as a disability, I see it as a setback.

Interviewer: Does anyone else see themselves as disabled?

Tina: Yes, it's not the same in the world as for hearing people, so if it's good for the image, it's fine by me.

Janet to Jeremy: Do you see it as an insult? Are you ashamed? Are you not proud of being deaf?

Jeremy: No, I am saying I don't see it as a disability. I've never gone to anyone and said, 'Please help me, please help me, I'm deaf'.

Interviewer: Who feels disabled?

Tina: I admit I am disabled but it feels wrong – what does disabled mean, like not being able to do something, like being in a wheelchair?

Janet: I have a disability, because I haven't got first-class communication, because I can't hear, but it's not the right word, disabled means incapable.

Amanda: We're not really disabled, we can move, the sign means can't move.

Interviewer: Do you see yourselves as a disabled group or like an ethnic minority group with your own way of life, sign language and part of Deaf culture, or do you see yourselves as disadvantaged?

Amanda: I feel I belong to the Deaf group.

Interviewer: But as part of a group of disabled people?

Amanda: That's hard to say.

Tina: I tell people I'm Deaf, not disabled. At the same time I think of myself as part of a Deaf group. I do see myself as disabled, though, because I can't use the telephone. I'm not sure about Deaf culture.

Interviewer: What is meant by Deaf culture?

Tina: Deaf Club, Deaf way of life, the language and the history.

Interviewer: Do you feel part of that?

Tina: Yes, I consider myself part of that. All my friends are deaf, so that's where I belong.

Janet: I recognise myself as part of a disabled group. I think if I dissociated myself from them it would be condescending and snobbish about it to someone who was more disabled.

The discussion threw up a number of interesting points, which also arise in discussion with the Deaf community in general. The first concerns whether being a linguistic and cultural minority group precluded a person from being disabled. For a number of the group not being able to use the telephone or communicate easily by speech was disabling. A further concern was the impact on other disabled groups of Deaf people accepting or rejecting the disabled label. One felt that its acceptance was an insult to other disabled people who had different requirements from himself, and felt he might be being used politically. Others felt that rejection of the

Table 7.7. *Young people's and parents' perception of newspaper reading habits*

	Parents' perception		
	Includes broadsheets	Tabloids only	Does not read
Young people's perception			
Includes broadsheets	5	4	0
Tabloids only	11	33	6
Rarely/never reads	0	2	0

disabled label might be oppressive or discriminatory against disabled people in general, a view strongly argued by Finkelstein (1991). Such issues are clearly not simple and were not easily discussed in the interview situation. It was in the group context that the young people felt happier to develop and express their ideas in this area.

POLITICS AND RELIGION

Beyond their understanding of deaf issues, we were also concerned with the appreciation that the young people had of world affairs, political ideas, and social issues. Access to much of this information is provided through the media, so first we looked at whether they had access to TV or newspapers. All of them could answer the question as to whether they read newspapers and only one said they never did and only one said they rarely did. Of the remainder, 50 (82%) read the popular press only, three (5%) the broadsheets only, and six (10%) both. The vast majority reading the papers said they read a mixture of items, although two claimed to look only at sport and two to read only for human interest stories. For interest, we compared this with the parents' accounts of the newspapers read by the young people, shown in Table 7.7. This seems to indicate a relatively consistent relationship, and with parents seeing rather more as reading broadsheets, and also rather more as not reading the papers at all. It will be remembered that the parents were also asked about the young people's reading ability, and this showed a consistent relationship with accounts of papers read, although one would not necessarily expect a direct matching.

Competence in reading does not necessarily mean a person does read the papers. Of the two who reported they never or rarely read the papers, one was seen as an adequate and the other as a competent reader. Of the 50 who said they read the tabloid press, six were seen as poor readers, 28 as adequate readers and 16 as competent readers. Of the nine who included broadsheets in the newspaper reading, eight were seen as competent readers and one as adequate. Therefore, nearly all those reading broadsheets were seen by their parents as competent readers and none were seen as poor readers. Overall, these data seem to indicate some access to the media via newspapers.

Most of them (59) had access to a television and all except one of these watched it. Of these, 35 (60%) watched programmes designed for deaf people or subtitled programmes only. The other 23 (40%) included other programmes and three of these claimed never to watch specialist deaf programmes or use subtitles.

Therefore, superficially, the young people would seem to have some access to news media, although it should be noted that those not included in the analysis of young people's interviews included a higher proportion of young people with difficulty in reading and who did not read newspapers.

To get some indication of their participation in politics, we asked whether they voted in the last election. Of the 57 answering this question and who were eligible to vote, 42 (74%) had voted and 15 (26%) had not. This was consistent with voting figures for the population as a whole, where 75% voted. Of those voting, one-third (14) voted in the way suggested to them by their parents and two-thirds (28) had decided for themselves.

To probe political awareness further, the young people were asked their opinions on a number of issues in the general area of current events. Our aim was not to arrive at definitive statements about the political or social views of deaf young people; firstly, because of the high proportion (one-third) who took their views directly from their parents in matters such as voting; and secondly, because this often would not have been possible, as the answers they gave often expressed a complex view not coming down on one side or the other. Rather, we were interested to establish which topics concerned and interested the young people and also those they knew little about. The subject was introduced by asking:

'I would like to ask your opinion on some matters' and then various statements were made. At the time of the interviews, Margaret Thatcher was Prime Minister and Neil Kinnock leader of the opposition. (The difference between asking such questions in BSL and in English is discussed in Appendix III) Responses were classified into 'complex', 'simple' and 'not answered'. The distinction between these categories is described in Chapter 1. Table 7.8 shows those giving complex answers to the state-

Table 7.8. *Answers to political and social questions*

		Complex answers (%)	Not answered (%)
F.	All policeman should have guns	46	11
L.	Abortion is a woman's decision	43	28
M.	Hanging should be brought back	34	10
E.	Woman should not go to work but stay at home	33	5
G.	Violence on television makes violence in real life worse	28	15
K.	Rape is a serious crime	26	7
A.	Margaret Thatcher is a good Prime Minister	26	5
I.	The British Army should come out of Ireland	25	13
H.	It is bad for couples to live together without getting married	20	7
N.	It is all right for gay people to live together	20	6
B.	Neil Kinnock could be a better Prime Minister	18	7
D.	Black people should rule South Africa	18	30
J.	Most people who are out of work are too lazy to look for work	18	20
C.	Nuclear power is safe to make	10	31

ments and those who could not answer or to whom the question was not put. The letter indicates the position of each statement on the presentation.

The questions that called forth the most complex responses were those on law and order (police and hanging) and women's issues (abortion, women working and rape). Those that received the fewest complex answers were those on nuclear power, unemployment, South Africa and Kinnock. While it is the case that the issues that received the fewest complex answers were likely to be those that were the most difficult to answer, for example those on South Africa, nuclear power and unemployment, the converse is not the case. Some questions that received proportionally high numbers of complex answers were also questions that were difficult to answer. An obvious one is the question concerning abortion, for while 43% of the answers were complex, 28% were unable to provide an opinion. The same applies in a less dramatic way to the questions on TV violence and Ireland.

In our interviews with the young people, we also focused on a particular topical issue: their understanding of HIV and AIDS. This was found to be an area in which the young people felt particularly well informed. Six could not answer a question about AIDS and two said they knew nothing about it. However, the remaining 53 (87%) felt well informed and most had obtained information from a number of sources. This is probably due to general media coverage of the topic plus the attention given to providing access to information by the Deaf organisations, notably the British Deaf Association. Some had felt almost overwhelmed by the publicity.

I have had it from See Hear (the BBC magazine programme for deaf viewers), newspapers, leaflets through the door, mother, father, everyone. I've heard so much about it, it's coming out of my ears. The Mission had a doctor explain it with an interpreter – that was very good.
Isabel, 21 years, SSE

Most had a non-condemning attitude to people with AIDS.

They are just people. People who have got a problem they can't cure.
Malcolm, 22 years, oral

If I met someone I would act normally. They're not lepers, they are just unfortunate.
Jane, 20 years, oral

To address a further issue of concern with young people, we also asked if anyone had discussed drugs or glue sniffing with them, and of the 59 who could answer the question, 32 (54%) had discussed the issue with someone.

As well as politics, we were interested to find out their attitudes to religion. It has been suggested that in the past, because of the Church's involvement with deaf people, many deaf people were more likely to claim religious beliefs than hearing people (Lysons, 1979). When asked about church membership, 44 (72%) said they had no connection with the church at all, and no interest in religion, and five (8%) were regular church goers and believed in God. Five (8%) had been church attenders but no longer went, and three (5%) went to church but said they did not believe in God. A further four (7%) said they liked to discuss religious matters, two of these saying they did believe in some sort of God and two that they did not. This is markedly different and almost the reverse of a survey in the 1960s when 74% of the female deaf school leavers and 78% of the males attended church (Rodda, 1970), but probably reflects the changing times, rather than factors specific to deafness.

A FOCUS ON SPECIFIC GROUPS

In our discussion up to now we have focused on general characteristics of the sample as a whole, their attitudes to deafness, the world of Deaf people and political issues. However, in doing this we are aware of specific groups within the main sample who warrant special consideration, either because of their specific characteristics, or because they have not been part of the quantitative analysis. This includes those who do not consider their deafness to be a significant issue and live their lives in the hearing world and two groups that, for different reasons, have not been considered in the quantitative analysis, those from minority ethnic communities and those who could not be interviewed because of poor communication. There is also a further group, which we ourselves felt to be of special concern.

Living in the hearing world

Although this chapter has, in the main, focused on attitudes to deafness and relationships to the Deaf world, there was a small group who lived their lives within the hearing world. All those identified by their parents as having only hearing friends were in this group (12, 15%). Rather more of the deaf young people (22) had said that all their friends were hearing, but at other points in some of these interviews it was clear that they also had contact with deaf people. Not surprisingly, for all of this group their preferred communication was oral and they were, in general, those with the lesser hearing losses; ten of them (83%) were partially hearing or moderately deaf. Of the other two, one was severely deaf and one was profoundly deaf, although, because of physical disabilities, he had been educated in a special unit for most of his school career and was in the group with limited language skills. (Therefore, he was not interviewed in the young people's interviews, the only one of this group, making a sample of eleven for some of the data reported here.) The group consisted of nine young men and three young women. Most of them had attended mainstream school at some time, four had been in mainstream schools throughout, five had attended mainstream and PHU's, and two had attended PHUs throughout.

In the interview, for which all had hearing notetakers, the interviewer felt that nine were at ease during the interview and with communicating through speech. These are comments from the interviewer's notes taken at the time.

> Throughout the interview, Ruth responded like a hearing person. () When I asked about communication with her parents, she said there was no physical difficulty and went on to talk about communication in the sense of how one approaches a subject in conversation, etc.

> Francis was very oral, so much so that if you used any visual cues they

appeared not to help at all. He spent a year at D... (college for deaf
people) yet does not know the finger-spelling alphabet.

For two of them, however, it was difficult. One of these, who was severely
deaf, had difficulty understanding speech, although he claimed it was
easier for him, saying:

> *I've seen sign language, but I think I am better at talking and listening.*
> *John, 22 years, oral*

The notes on his interview read:

> John's ability to lip read me was very poor. A lot of questions I had to
> repeat or show him the questions. His tenses are all in the present, even
> when talking about past incidents. This caused me some confusion as to
> whether he was talking about the past or the present.

The other young man who had difficulty communicating by speech found
many of the concepts very difficult. The notes on his interview suggest
problems in many areas: vocabulary, tense, 'as if' questions, describing
feelings, etc.

Of those who found it easy to communicate themselves, however, one
had difficulty in coping with an interviewer who was herself deaf. He spoke
very quickly and quietly and when asked to slow down said he did not like
meeting deaf people, as it inhibited him too much and made him unable to
relax.

Eight made extensive use of hearing aids, five wearing them all the time
and three most of the time, specifying they did not wear them in noisy
contexts. Three did not wear aids, as they felt better without them. One
commented:

> *At school I had to wear it. It must have helped me. The tutor at college*
> *made me wear it on placement, but I did not find it helpful. It made*
> *things louder but not clearer.*
> *Louise, 22 years, oral*

All of this group except one wished they were hearing, although for six it
was for purely functional reasons, such as getting a better job or hearing
announcements at stations. Ruth, though, when asked if she wished she
was hearing, said:

> *I wouldn't know how to cope. () I am proud to be deaf. It's a fault they*
> *can't change.*
> *Ruth, 19 years, oral*

The group included five of the young men who felt hearing partners to be ideal. The others did not answer the question (two) or felt other characteristics were more important to them than hearing loss (four). In discussing educational provision, most of the group favoured mainstream education (three), a variation on mainstream (three) or PHUs as the best option (two). None of this group saw schools for the deaf as the favoured option for deaf children, although three said that placement should depend on the need of the child. Most of this group (eight) expressed the view that while they had chosen to live their lives in the hearing world, they appreciated that others could make a different choice.

We ourselves felt that seven of the group were coping with the hearing world. We were concerned about the two who found the interview difficult, and a further two, one of whom is discussed in a later section (p. 214) and one of whom was the young man who described himself as having no friends.

Young people from minority ethnic groups

We were able to contact six of the 14 original families from minority ethnic groups and talk to four of the deaf young people, though the structured interview was not used. Research into deaf people from minority ethnic groups suggests that they are discriminated against in many areas – education, employment and provision of services (Sharma & Love, 1991). It is also suggested that they may not be accepted by the Deaf community. However, these issues were not apparent in the families we talked to. This was perhaps because all four of the young deaf people we were able to interview came from families who were part of the Asian community in a Midland city with a large Asian population. The families had all lived there for at least 20 years and were well established within the community. All the young people had attended the same residential school at secondary stage and all had maintained contact with friends from there. All could drive and two owned their own cars, which they used to visit their wide circle of friends. One contrasted his own experience with that of his hearing brother.

> *Deaf people are spread all over the country – they like to get together from all over the place and they meet in one place, but that is different in the hearing world. My brother does not know that many people in Wales and Scotland, but deaf people do and they meet quite regularly. So our parents worry a lot of the time, because we do all this travelling.*
> *Raj, 23 years, BSL*

Important in the lives of these particular young men was the local Deaf Club, which had an Asian section. The only complaint about this was the predominance of men attending the Club – about four out of every five members were male. Although it was a separate part of the Deaf Club, it seemed to bring white and Asian people together in a way that did not happen to these young men in the wider community.

In the Deaf Club the white and Asian people mix, we sometimes have parties together, but outside we are separate.

Ritesh, 24 years, BSL

Their apparent satisfaction with Deaf Club is at variance with the experience of many deaf people from minority ethnic groups. In reporting their study of this population, Sharma & Love (1991) comment:

Black deaf people felt their cultural identity was ignored. At times they felt overtly discriminated against, and some suffered racial abuse. Many respondents were too distressed to discuss the matter. Some white deaf groups were seen as defensive in not allowing black members to join them, or making black members feel uncomfortable if they attempted to become involved.

Most of this group insisted that the main issue for them was not being Asian but being deaf. In reporting this we do not want to suggest that there are no issues for Asian deaf young people. It is clear to us that the particular way in which this research developed meant that this group may not have been typical of the wider Asian population. There were more issues of concern for the parents, as we discuss in the next chapter.

Young people excluded from the quantitative analysis

It appeared he went through the motions of communicating without communicating

As was described in Chapter 1, of the 82 families involved at the parent interview stage, 14 of the young people were excluded from the analysis, because they did not have the communication skills necessary to be interviewed, or their interviews could not be adequately coded for analysis. Four young people were not interviewed, because of information given by their parents and a further four were visited but not interviewed. In the first instance the parents gave clear indications in their interviews, and advised us that it would not be possible to interview the young people. A description of Brian's communication by his mother is included in Chapter 2. Another mother said:

He communicates by gesture. The only thing he can say is 'Mam'. I've got him to say that.
Mother of Guy, 21 years, LLS

For a further four the interview had to be abandoned. Notes taken at the time may illustrate why.

Matthew is profoundly deaf with very limited communication – basic sign and occasional flashes of good fluid BSL features. He has a tendency to mouth words that are said to him simultaneously, as if echoing the person. He also tends to give responses that he thinks I want of him, e.g. negative facial expression plus 'You don't like flying do you?' gets the response 'No'. If it is 'Is your brother deaf?' it would be 'Yes' but likewise, 'Is your brother hearing?' it would also be 'Yes'. Otherwise, it's 'Yes' and 'No' apparently at random.

Interview with Matthew, 21 years, LLS, abandoned

Neil comes over as a cheerful, happy-go-lucky young lad who tends to think about the here and now, but this is perhaps because he finds it difficult to understand the concept of the future – or he might not really have had much of this kind of communication experience – or not have been exposed to this concept much. He had very little use of signs and gestures, and his speech pronunciation and even lip patterns were imprecise. At times it appeared he went through the motions of communicating without communicating. () What was horrendous was that he thought he was communicating with us and behaved as if he was able to do this. () Even when J... (notetaker) tried one question with Neil, such as, 'You went to four different schools; how old were you when you went to the first one – four, five, or six years? He responded, 'Twelve or thirteen, don't know'. () The whole interview was confusing. Even though I abandoned the schedule after the first page, it still lasted one and a half hours.

Interview with Neil, 20 years, LLS, abandoned

All these eight were described as having limited language skills. They were all male, five were classified as profoundly deaf, one as severely deaf and two as moderately deaf. Six of them, at the time of the second interview, had been labelled as having learning difficulties, and one as being physically disabled (cerebral palsy). At the time of their first interviews, when those in this group were aged three years six months to five years nine months, two were described as having disabilities other than deafness, one with a heart problem and the other with cerebral palsy. At the time of the first interview, four were described as having no expressive language, one had three words, one had one word and one was trying to speak. The other

(Neil, described above) is somewhat of an anomaly, as in the first interview when he was three years, nine months, he was reported as having 78 words. In this group he seemed the most able; he was the only one in work, having been retained in a small local firm after a job scheme placement there. He has passed the driving test and drives, although his mother commented that he would be unable to read the road signs. We wonder if in addition to his hearing loss, which was moderate, he had some specific language disorder.

In the group, two had attended schools for the deaf throughout, and one had attended a school for the deaf for the period for which information was available. Two had attended a combination of PHUs and schools for the deaf. The young man with cerebral palsy had initially attended a PHU, but had quickly been transferred to a school for the physically disabled and remained in this type of placement for the rest of his school career. One had started at PHUs but had later transferred to a Special Unit. At the time of the interviews, one was unemployed, three were in sheltered workshops, one was on a life skills course. One was on a job scheme, and was one of those who had been bullied at work (see Chapter 4), and one was employed. Work was a concern to the parents.

I went to see the careers officer.
Interviewer: What happened then?
Well, he just said he thought he would never get a job. I've seen the disabled officer at the Job Centre and he said he thought he'd never get a job.
Interviewer: Why?
He said, 'Well, it's all speed now' and with people like him, you've got to show him, because you can't talk to him. You've got to show him and I suppose you'd have to stay with him for a bit, because, you know, to see if he could do it right and they just haven't got the time.
Mother of Brian, 22 years, LLS

He'll always need a lot of help. He just comes home and sits. He expects to be taken out. We thought maybe farming and arranged for him to help a friend, but it's too high tech, there's too much machinery. I am plugging gardening now, but he won't dig, he's not interested.
Mother of Tony, 22 years, LLS

Parents tended to perceive them as vulnerable and immature, particularly in sexual matters, and saw little hope of them becoming independent.

He worries me every time he goes into H... I'm worried about the road. I'm worried he's not going to be looking. Will he forget? All the time,

constantly. I'm worried if anybody talks to him. I've told him never to go walking with anybody or get into anybody's car. He wouldn't, but he is so vulnerable. Physically he wouldn't be able to defend himself at all.
Mother of Matthew, 21 years, LLS

His limited background knowledge of things makes him immature.
Mother of Neil, 20 years, LLS

He's mature in body but not in mind, he's still at the giggly stage. He knows he's got to be married, I've taught him that, because I don't want him to touch anybody.
Mother of Tony, 22 years, LLS

He'll say he doesn't want a girlfriend. He says he's going to stop with me at home. The relationship we have now is not healthy. It's too much with me. I do worry about it a lot this last couple of years. He should be going out.
Mother of Matthew, 21 years, LLS

I think he would like to have more independence, but it would be difficult for him to go and live elsewhere.
Mother of Neil, 20 years, LLS

Inevitably, these concerns lead to general worries about the future.

Interviewer: What do you worry about?
His future as a whole. Everything. What is going to happen to him. I know how way behind he is. As Matthew stands now, he is causing me a lot of worry.
Mother of Matthew, 21 years, LLS

While this chapter started by considering the perspective of the young people themselves on their deafness, here we describe a group for whom the discussion must be via other reports. Already, through their lack of language they have little voice; to omit them here would be to marginalise them even further. Some seemed to be in this group because they had been simply denied the opportunity to develop language and to participate in the events around them. The question remains as to whether this group had fundamental learning difficulties, which combined with their deafness had led to poor language skills, or whether other factors in addition to their deafness had led to their poor language development and the label of learning difficulties has been consequent upon this.

He blushed and smiled a lot when he did not understand the questions

A further six were interviewed, but their responses were not used in the quantitative analysis. In two instances, the replies were such that we did not attempt to code them and in the other four we coded the responses, but more than 20% of the interview could not be coded (21–34%). This in itself made it difficult to use the analysis, but it also threw some doubts on some of the responses that had been coded. For example, many of the other answers were 'yes' or 'no' and it was not always clear that the question had been understood.

Excerpts extracted from notes made immediately after the interview may make this clearer.

On Edward's arrival, Edward's mother told him to put on his hearing aids and said to me on one side that it would be very interesting to see if I could get anything out of him. Once on our own it became very clear that Edward had very little idea why we were there and I had to prompt him heavily throughout the interview. He has no knowledge of sign language but he uses gesture and speech. His command of spoken English is very poor, considering he says he is able to function without his hearing aids when socialising at the welfare club, playing football, etc. He blushed and smiled a lot when he did not understand the questions.
Interview with Edward, 23 years, oral, not coded

SSE used throughout. Great difficulty in comprehension. Jenny was only able to cope with questions about the present that related to herself. Could not cope with could, would, wish, suppose questions.
Interview with Jenny, 19 years, SSE, coded but not used; 43 of 110 categories (39%) uncodable

It was very difficult for me to communicate with Dennis, because of Dennis's lack of experience in handling questions such as those on the interview schedule. () His technique of answering a question when he did not really understand what was being asked of him was to respond, 'Some', Sometimes', 'Same', 'Some the same' and on these occasions even if we prompted Dennis it was quite hard to get his thoughts on the subject. Dennis gave the impression that he has been resigned to not following what's going on around him, not really bothering to try and find out and that his family did not really keep him informed at times. () One can see from the interview that he became most responsive on issues directly related to him, in the here and now.

Dennis, 19 years, BSL, coded but not used; 35 of 110 categories (32%) uncodable

For this group the problem seemed to be not simply a difficulty with language, but unfamiliarity with a situation in which they were asked for their views, and an acquired tendency to say, 'Yes' or 'No' or 'Maybe' when they did not understand. Many of the group had little communication within their own families. For example, the interviewer's notes on Jean (22 years, SSE) describe this.

> Her comprehension of questions was not very good, but I feel this was partly due to lack of real communication at home and not having positive experiences in relation to her own peer group. At times, because of the nature of the questions, she asked, 'How do you know that?' as if I knew something about her in order to ask that question, e.g. 'Did your mother and father discuss personal matters with you?'

Ann, a BSL user, 21 years old, had been excluded from many family events. She did not know why her mother and father had split up; the first she knew of her mother's remarriage was when her stepfather moved in. She was working in a shop, a job she did not like, because it was arranged for her as a YTS scheme and she had stayed on. She would have preferred to work in the local electronics factory. Although she had a boyfriend, and planned to go and live with him, she said she knew little about sex – her mother had told her nothing; she had learnt some from school and some from books. She seemed to have little contact with her family, although she lived with them. At first she said:

> I eat with the family but I don't join in any talk; after dinner I go to my room and watch TV.

Later she said that often in fact she did not eat with the family, but cooked for herself and took it to her room. She had some contact with other deaf people; there was a deaf young woman living locally whom she met occasionally and her boyfriend visited when he could, although she had met him first at school and he lived some distance away.

Although this group is not included in the quantitative results, quotes from their interviews are included in the body of the text. We were able to make the decision about their preferred communication. Three of them were BSL users, two preferred SSE, and one was oral. Four of this group were classified as profoundly deaf and two as severely deaf. Two had visual difficulties in addition to their deafness, but none of the others were described as having other disabilities.

Table 7.9. *Negative self evaluations given by deaf young people*

	Number	%
None	19	31
One	28	46
Two	7	11
Three	4	7
Four	2	3
Five	1	2

Cause for concern

Better dead than deaf

In our interviews, over half the young people indicated that they accepted their deafness, and it was an integral part of their lives. However, there was a group that caused us great concern. These were those young people with very low self esteem. Six particular questions from the schedule seemed to be good indicators of self esteem and we use them to identify this group.

Are you a happy or sad person?
Are you confident or not very confident?
Do you like yourself?
Do you ever feel proud of yourself?
Do you ever feel sorry for yourself?
Are there any things about yourself that you do not like and wish to change? (We excluded concrete changes such as 'my hair' or wishing to be slimmer.)

Negative responses to these were taken to be feeling a sad person, feeling not very confident, not liking oneself, not feeling proud of oneself, feeling sorry for oneself and wanting to change oneself. They had to be definite responses; answers that were qualified in some way or spoke of 'sometimes' or 'it varies' would be coded differently. Occasionally it was a matter for interpretation. The quote at the beginning of this chapter, from Carol, which includes the words, 'I am a terrible person' would not be classed as a negative response because of the context and the way in which it was conveyed. The proportion giving negative answers to this group of questions is shown in Table 7.9.

About two-thirds of the sample (42/61, 69%) gave negative responses to at least one question. However, we decided that those giving more than half negative responses, i.e. three or more, seemed cause for concern. This was the case for one in nine (11%) of the total sample, although even this is probably an underestimate. These were difficult questions for some to answer. For each question there were a number who could not understand the question or formulate a response. There were 19 who could not answer one of the questions, ten who could not answer two and five who could not answer three. Therefore, less than half the sample (27/61) could answer all the questions. Those who had difficulty with one or more questions are likely to be under-represented here. It may be that a similar proportion of hearing young people would present the same degree of negative evaluation of themselves. However, we found that to focus on the seven young people who gave negative answers to three or more of the questions was itself revealing, particularly in considering the factors associated with this. We have decided to drop names (pseudonyms) for this section to prevent any possibility of recognition, particularly within families.

Their feelings of lack of self worth were very strong. The most dramatic was a deaf youth who three times in his interview commented that it would be better to be dead than deaf. He also said:

I never like what I am, I feel a bad character, I wish I was not alive. I've had a lot of pressure put on me, I'm always on my own, I talk to myself.

Others said:

I feel angry inside. I want to be perfect like other people.

I feel sad, boring, I have nothing to talk about. ( ) I don't feel confident. I want to feel better. I want to feel more confident, I want to be a better signer so I can communicate more.

My body, my face and the inside of me, I do not like it.

I don't like myself and nobody likes me. ( ) I feel sad, I feel nobody, I can't talk.

I am a sad person most of the time. I often feel hurt but I keep my feelings to myself.

Interestingly, a factor that was common to most of these young people was the report of serious teasing at work or school, and there was evidence of this for six out of the seven.

The reasons that this group should feel so negatively about themselves were complex, and different for different young people. Looking at the basic information, no clear factors emerge. There were five males and two females. They were educated in a range of settings and employed in a range of work situations. Three were oral, three BSL users and one used SSE. Five were severely deaf and two moderately deaf. They were no more likely than the rest of the sample to come from homes where the marriage had broken up or was experiencing difficulties. However, in considering the young people and their families, there did seem to be some common factors, which we speculate on here. In one case, however, we should point out that an additional contributory factor was likely to be significant physical abuse by the father over a number of years.

Five of the young people were among that group that wished they were hearing.

> *I wish I was born hearing. () Life would be different. I would have a lot of hearing friends, I would have a proper job.*

> *I don't mind being deaf, but if I was hearing I would have more friends.*

> *Life would be better, I'd be cleverer. It would be easier with people. I'd hear music, get a better education.*

The mother of another commented:

> *He doesn't want to know about being deaf. I mean, we went through a big phase where he wasn't deaf in his eyes. All right, he wore his hearing aids, but say, 'You are deaf' and he got stroppy with you.*

Two of the group expressed feelings of not belonging with deaf people, although in both cases it was seen as a loss. Both these two wished they were hearing and both were oral.

> *Last year I went to a party. All the deaf people could sign. I couldn't. I felt left out and I cried. I couldn't understand without voice.*

> *Interviewer: Have you seen deaf people using sign language?*
> *Yes, in Lourdes, France. There were deaf handicapped using sign language. I felt different, I felt more with them than with myself, signing with them. () In the group, I talked to deaf people. It was like being back at school, talking to deaf people, it felt good. I was pleased to be with deaf people, coming away I felt bad about myself.*

This rejection of deafness seemed to have its roots, in part, in the family and in particular in an emphasis on normality and a rejection of things to do with deafness. Three of the parents expressed the desirability of normality throughout their interviews using expression such as, 'She was going to marry somebody normal, which we knew as a mixed marriage would not work anyway'; 'Children that are normal don't accept the handicapped'; 'If he'd had his normal hearing he would be...'.

The young people in these families also emphasised the desirability of normality.

When I was young they wanted me to be like a normal person, speak very well. They did not want me to sign, because my speech would go bad.

People don't understand odd people. They don't want deaf people if they aren't normal. It makes me say I don't want to be deaf.

I didn't feel deaf before I was seven – I was normal.

In addition, in some families there seemed to be a rejection of deafness itself. One young person commented:

My parents are nice to my brother and sister (hearing). They argue with me. They say they don't like deaf people.

In other families there was a rejection of aspects of deaf people's lives. Five of the families were seen by their sons or daughters to be opposed to the use of sign language, and a further one to have been opposed until very recently. This does not in all cases agree with the parental account of the situation, but was the young person's perception.

A BSL user said:

My father and mother want me, but not signing. I ask them why they don't want me to sign; they say they want me to improve my speech, but that's impossible.

And her mother confirmed this in saying:

We wanted her to talk as far as possible.

In the oral young people, opposition to signing was often to endorse normality.

My parents don't like signing, they think I should use lip reading.

The mother here spoke of advice she would give to parents of newly diagnosed deaf children.

The first thing is to make sure you get them to talk as normally as you can. I swear the majority of them can talk. Get their speech as near to normal as possible, it helps you and it helps them.

And another mother of an oral young person said:

> *They did a lot of sign language which I didn't agree with. Quite a bit of oral, but I mean obviously fell back on the sign language which, to be honest, I don't know whether this is right or wrong, I have never let him use it. () I let him use whatever means he wanted to communicate, but not signing.*

In three of the families the young deaf person was discouraged from using subtitles, even though they wanted to.

> *I told my mother I would like teletext but she said it was too much money.*

> *My father chooses what television programmes we watch. He doesn't let me watch the subtitled ones if he doesn't want to watch them. If I try to watch See Hear my father either turns it off or switches channels. I have a TV in my room, but I am not allowed to watch it, because of the cost of the electricity.*

> *If there are any programmes with sign language, my mother switches them off.*

In a further case, the family had bought teletext television, but the young person themselves had rejected it. He said:

> *We have teletext but we don't use. I don't feel happy using it. I lip read.*
> *Interviewer: What do you do if you can't see the face?*
> *I turn it up.*
> *Interviewer: Does this make it hard for you?*
> *Yes.*

His father commented:

> *I think it is because he won't have the teletext on and we don't have the sound up high especially for him, because I think we have got teletext television for him and we got that purposely; he just won't have it.*
> *Interviewer: Why do you think that is?*
> *I think it takes away the being normal. He has got to be normal all the time.*

In three of the families the young person was discouraged from going to Deaf Club despite the fact that they wanted to go.

> *If I had gone to Deaf Club that would have helped me make more friends and be more confident. () My mother and father held me back*

three years. Now I am trying to catch up. I asked first if I could go to the Deaf Mission. ( ) I told my cousin I wanted to see deaf people and make friends but my mother and father kept me in prison at home. My cousin helped me; he telephoned my mother and said, 'Please take...to Deaf Club to make friends and meet deaf people.

I went to Deaf Club with people from my school. Then my Mum said no more Deaf Club so I stopped.
Interviewer: Why did your Mum and Dad stop you going to Deaf Club? They said it was a long way.
Interviewer: Did you want to carry on going?
Yes.

I want to go to Deaf Club but it's hard to get there and I get home late. I wanted to go on the bus but there is no bus back so my father said 'No'. He wouldn't come and pick me up, I don't know why.

In addition to this, there was a disappointment in two of the families, where the parents simply felt disappointed in their young people.

I expected better things of him. That sounds bigheaded but yes, I am disappointed.

The teachers years ago used to say, 'Oh, she has got a good brain'. Yes, I thought, but she's encased in a useless body with it.

In two families, the deafness had been a result of rubella and the parents had considered abortion.

I had rubella, I should have had an abortion.

I am a great believer in it (abortion). Even now sex is casual, every baby should be wanted, so erase it if it is not. I wouldn't have brought...into the world to be like she is. ( ) Don't bring someone into the world if you know you've had German measles, honestly. Thank God you don't get many deaf kids.

Both the young people were aware of their parents' feelings.

Mother told me she would have aborted me if she had known about German measles.
Interviewer: What do you feel about that?
Yes, I agree about handicapped being aborted.
Interviewer: Deaf as well?
Yes.

In all of the families we have described except one, at least three of the following five characteristics have been described in the reports of the young people: emphasis on normality or explicit rejection of deafness, rejection of sign language, rejection of Deaf Club, rejection of teletext, a view that abortion is appropriate for cases of deafness. It seems to us that these were significant factors. There is of course a danger here; we could be asserting that such factors cause low self esteem, when all we can say is that when we look at young people with low self esteem, these elements are likely to be present.

We have referred to the one young person who does not fit easily here. He was a young man whose family accepted sign language, were very positive in their attitude to him and whose life seemed relatively problem-free. However, he himself had a very low opinion of himself, was constantly feeling he should do better, and felt unliked and unhappy. We suspect that this young man was probably suffering from some form of depression, not arising in a clear way from his immediate situation.

THE EFFECT OF DEAFNESS ON THE FAMILY

I've never thought about it being better for my father and mother

In the last section we indicated that some reasons for concern may lie in parental attitudes and we go on to look at the parents' views in more detail in the next chapter, but here we consider whether the young people felt their deafness had made any difference to their parents' lives. The young people were asked what effect their deafness had on their families and in particular for their parents. They were given the opportunity to comment on possible positive and negative consequences.

> Q29. *Do you think any of your family have suffered because you are deaf?*
> Q30. *Do you think life has been any better for any of your family because you are deaf?*

This was a difficult topic to ask about, and the questions were often omitted, either because the interviewer did not feel it appropriate to ask them in the particular circumstances or because the young person did not seem likely to understand the question. Both questions were omitted in 18 interviews, and in a further two where they were asked, it seemed that the young person had not understood the question. For question 30, the answer was sometimes derived from the answer to question 29. A further three answered the negative question but could not understand the positive one. Nearly a third of those answering Q 29 felt the deafness had made no negative difference (12/41, 29%). The most common description of difference in the others was to say that their parents had been upset when they were babies but not now (12/41, 29%). Other responses were additional worry (four), effect on family relationships including marriage breakup (three), difficulties around communication (two) and the number of decisions that needed to be made (two).

> *Yes, because they had to make a lot of decisions – which school I should go to, which hearing aid, whether to use speech or not.*
> *Tina, 18 years, oral*

Four young people, although they understood the question, felt they did not know the answer, one of them adding, 'I've never asked'.

The question as to whether the deafness had had a positive effect on the family was a difficult question, and three commented on this fact.

> *It's a difficult question, only they could really know.*
> *Tina, 18 years, oral*

> *I've never thought about that.*
> *Darren, 22 years, BSL*

> *I've never thought about it being better for my mother and father.*
> *Paula, 24 years, BSL*

A further three said they did not know. Over half (21/38) could think of no positive consequence for the family and a further six qualified this further by saying that there was no positive effect and that the only consequences were negative. The majority answering (27/38, 71%) saw no positive effect for the family at all. Five did suggest positive consequences, which included:

> *I don't think it has been better – maybe it is more rewarding in some ways because I have this disability. I hate saying this, but they are probably proud to have proved to people that I have coped just as well as other children. I think this has made a difference.*
> *Ruth, 19 years, oral*

> *They have met a lot of other parents of deaf children.*
> *Christine, 21 years, SSE*

> *It has been interesting for them.*
> *Paula, 24 years, BSL*

Our family relationships are better.
Shaun, 21 years, BSL

It has made my mother a better mother.
Zoe, 19 years, BSL

DEAFNESS AND YOUNG PEOPLE

In this chapter we have seen a diversity of experience of deafness for the young people. At the beginning we suggested that people might be concerned with identification with the hearing world or with the deaf world. In fact these strong identifications have emerged rarely. Most of the deaf young people lived in both and took a moderate position on this. While most accepted they were deaf and many saw it as an integral part of their identity, few talked of being proud to be deaf and strongly identifying with the Deaf community, although a significant number spent most of their social life with other deaf people. Likewise, although a small group chose to live their lives exclusively in the hearing world, only a minority minimised the consequences of their deafness and almost all of these had minor hearing losses.

CHAPTER EIGHT

The family and the young deaf person

Because of the deafness () we've organised things that we'd never have done, we've been to places we'd never have gone to, we've done things we'd never have done.
Mother of Veronica, 21 years, SSE

A deaf person alters the lives of everyone in a home; it's a big big disturbance in everything you do.
Mother of Colin, 24 years, BSL

For a hearing family to have a deaf son or daughter has consequences for the private and the public life of the family. Within the family, communication cannot be taken for granted in the way that it is where all the members are hearing or all the members are deaf. This has secondary effects for individual family members and for relationships within the family. Within society, the family becomes a focus of special attention, from doctors, educationalists and other professionals. The family is treated differently and thus can become different. Moreover, society is poorly adapted to meet the needs of deaf people in many ways, including communication and access to information, which creates further issues for the family. In this chapter we address many of the themes developed earlier in the book, but focus on their impact on the family. We start by considering the way in which the young deaf people are perceived by their parents and how this affects the relationship between them. We then look at the effect of deafness on relationships within the family and the effect the parents feel it has had on their own lives.

Table 8.1. *The personality of the young deaf people as described by their parents*

	Yes		Varies		No	
	Number	%	Number	%	Number	%
Calm	35	43	15	18	32	39
Anxious	29	35	11	13	42	51
Easily bored	43	52	4	5	35	43
Affectionate	51	62	10	12	21	27
Generally happy	51	62	23	28	8	10
Bad tempered	26	32	11	13	45	55
Aggressive	14	17	4	5	64	78

FROM CHILD TO ADULT – THE PARENTS' PERSPECTIVE

Continuity and consistency

In the last chapter, we examined how the deaf young people saw themselves. In this section, we look at how they were seen by their parents, whether there were any perceived consistent personality traits and, if so, whether these had consequences for family relationships. We also examine whether any childhood behaviours correlated with behaviour now.

The assessments of personality given by the parents is shown in Table 8.1. Our purpose in including these is not because we have a belief in these measures, or endorse the notion of such personality attributes, rather, it is to illustrate numerically the parents' perceptions of their sons and daughters. Overall, the view is positive, with no indications in these characteristics of a specific deaf personality. This view was endorsed by some of the parents in the interviews.

It (life) would have been a little bit calmer and not so frustrating. That's something we don't know, isn't it? I don't think it would have been so much different. He would still have had a lot of those characteristics. They were in his makeup and the deafness wouldn't have made much difference anyway.
Father of Alistair, 21 years, oral

We examined these data to see how consistent young people's and parental reports were for the categories that were assessed in both interviews. While agreement was not total and not statistically significant, most of the disagreements were accounted for by either the parent or young person

Table 8.2. *The relationship between temper tantrums as a child and personality now*

	Many tantrums	Few tantrums
Happy	27	24
Varies	20	3
Unhappy	7	1
Not easily bored	16	19
Varies	3	1
Easily bored	35	8

being specific about a category and the other describing it in a way that was classified as 'varies'. In general, the young person made more use of the variable category. Total disagreements, where one said 'happy' and one said 'unhappy' were 5/54 (9%) and for 'calm' or 'not calm', 7/46 (15%).

We also looked to see whether any of the later personality characteristics related to earlier behaviours, and we considered the information on temper tantrums from the interview when the young people were children (see Table 8.2). Although temper tantrums as a child did not show a significant relationship with any of the personality characteristics described by the young people themselves, they did show a significant relationship with two of the characteristics described by their parents. Those who were described as not happy or varying between happy and unhappy were significantly more likely to have had many temper tantrums as a child, while those who were describes as happy were almost evenly split between many and few temper tantrums ($\chi^2 = 10.03$ $p < 0.01$). Similarly, those who were described as easily bored were significantly more likely to have had many tantrums as a child ($\chi^2 = 11.031$ $p > 0.01$)

A deaf personality?

As described in the previous chapter, within the literature on deafness there have been suggestions that there is a typical deaf personality, usually described in a negative way. In our consideration of personality characteristics, there have been no indications of this. However, we specifically considered the allegations that have been made in the literature that deaf people are immature and egocentric. The question about immaturity was asked in the context of the extent to which parents felt their son or daughter had achieved independence. Egocentricity was derived from the answers to a number of questions in the schedules. In addition, we asked two specific questions about whether the young person would admit when

Table 8.3. *Egocentricity and immaturity as perceived by the parents*

	Yes		Varies		No	
	Number	%	Number	%	Number	%
Immature	40	49	2	2	40	49
Egocentric	35	43	2	2	45	55
Will admit when in the wrong	29	35	27	33	26	32
Will take a joke against self	36	44	15	18	31	38

in the wrong, and whether they could take a joke against themselves. Table 8.3 shows the extent to which the parents attributed these characteristics to their sons and daughters.

The concept of immaturity may have been inflated by those with limited language skills, as all eight were perceived as immature. If these are removed, the proportions are: mature 40 (54%), immature 32 (43%), varies 2 (3%). For the other characteristics, those with limited communication skills were distributed throughout the other categories, although more were seen as egocentric, unable to take a joke, unable to admit when in the wrong, than otherwise.

Often the perception of egocentricity arose from lack of understanding on the part of the young person.

It's very hard to make him see the subtleties that we have. Automatically it doesn't happen. He won't say, 'I know it's awfully inconvenient, but do you think...Just this once, please'; it's 'Now Mum, get me out, get me out of bed, take me to work'.
Mother of Darren, 22 years, BSL

I think they are self-centred. He still is. I mean now and again I have to jolt him and say – well there is somebody else. I mean I jolted him even the other week; I said, 'It is all because you are thinking of you, Wayne, think of other people. Don't you think we have problems as well? We have had a lot of problems' so I reeled them off to him. So I says, 'There you are, you see, but we are still here, we have got over them, and you will get over yours'.
Mother of Wayne, 21 years, oral

In many respects the above examples seem to have much in common with ordinary teenage behaviour. However, there were a small number of instances where attitudes and expectations of parents seemed somewhat different. Some of the young people made unreasonable demands, because they assumed competence or knowledge in people that was not there, usually because they perceived their hearing parents as having knowledge and understanding of the world that they did not have. This mother describes how her daughter expected her to know about passports, although the mother had never been abroad.

She asked me to fill it in, but I said, 'no, you fill it in. You can ask me questions about it but I can't fill it in in my own handwriting, you have got to do it'. And she just had to have another signature, somebody like a Justice or whatever, and I just said, 'Go and ask' because I had never filled in a passport thing in my life. And I said, 'Ask people who have been abroad before and then they will tell you how to go about it', but she couldn't understand why I didn't know. I couldn't get through to her. It was the same as things on the television, discovery things or whatever, she keeps on saying 'how?' 'what for?', you know, 'what's it about?' and when I said I didn't know she got upset as if I should know.
Mother of Rachel, 22 years, BSL

As Rachel's mother indicated, the egocentricity was not a direct consequence of deafness, but it occurred in some of the young people as a secondary consequence, because they did not have the same information available to them as would be expected of a hearing young person of the same age.

With perceptions of immaturity also, parents were likely to attribute this to lack of knowledge of the world, and suggested that as their sons and daughters became more experienced they became more able to cope.

Well, he is getting more and more mature. It is coming on in leaps and bounds. Where he has been very behind, and still is to a degree, in a lot of things, but he is coming on in leaps and bounds. Buying the house has been a tremendous jump for him and a tremendous worry, but it has been ever so good.
Mother of Colin, 24 years, BSL

They are not as grown up at her age as a normal 21 year old is. They are about, what, three years behind, and I think that is with all deaf children whatever age they are, they are not as grown up as what a normal hearing.
Interviewer: *Why do you think that is?*
Well, let's face it. They miss out a lot on life, don't they, really?
Mother of Sharon, 21 years, BSL

An issue, which was raised spontaneously by a number of parents and seems relevant here, was the view that the deaf young person was mean or especially cautious with money. Although we did not ask about this specifically, this suggestion was made in a significant number of interviews. Of the parents (42) who spontaneously mentioned attitude to money, nearly three-quarters (31, 74%) described their sons and daughters as being particularly careful with money.

> *He's all right at looking after his money. He always makes sure he gives over the right amount for an article; he doesn't like giving the wrong amount. ( ) We don't know why this is, and wonder if all deaf people do it.*
> *Father of Shaun, 21 years, BSL*

> *Mother: Oh she will soon tell you if she is short changed.*
> *( )*
> *Father: Dead shrewd to the point of meanness.*
> *Mother: I mean, she is on piece work and she knows the money she has got due to her on a Friday.*
> *Father: She has got a notebook.*
> *Mother: She writes it all down.*
> *Parents of Sharon, 21 years, BSL*

> *He's not too bad at clinging onto money. He knows what money is.*
> *Father of Clive, 20 years, BSL*

We were surprised that this should emerge in the interviews. It was not something we ourselves had experienced and we had not asked specifically about it in the interview. One interpretation of the finding would be to say that a certain proportion of young people are very careful with money. We would not agree with this, as most of the parents we spoke to were making comparisons with siblings and other young people that they knew, and it was in this context that the young people were seen as being mean. Because it was raised so often, we did feel that there was an issue here, and there seemed to be a number of elements that came together. Firstly, there was the age at which the interviews were carried out, which was when there was a specific concern with money, as the young people were becoming financially independent of their parents, through starting work or college or drawing unemployment benefit. Moreover, many of them were embarking on considering large purchases for the first time, such as a house or car. Secondly, many of the young people needed specific guidance or information about managing money, which usually came from their parents. Such information is often acquired incidentally by hearing young people from the media, from advertisements or television programmes or the like, and many discuss these things with their friends. Hearing people have easy access to building societies and banks, which are only too enthusiastic to discuss financial matters. Such information was more difficult for deaf young people to access. We wondered if, although financial affairs were difficult, they constituted an area where young people could assert their independence, take control, manage and plan their money. It may be that exclusion from the dominant society means there are few of these areas, and the appearance of caution is a demonstration of developing autonomy.

In terms of personality, though, most of the information we have indicates that over half of the group were not seen as particularly immature or egocentric. Over half of them would admit when they were in the wrong at least some of the time, and most could take a joke against themselves. Where they were seen as having negative attributes, this could be seen not as an irrevocable consequence of their deafness, but as a lack of awareness, due to limited information received, or an attempt to manage in a world for which they were not fully prepared. Full access to communication could thus change this.

Some parents saw a lack of access to the hearing world as having positive rather than negative consequences.

She is not devious in any way, because she has not learnt to be devious. She is not deceitful, because she does not know about deceitfulness. She's straightforward, honest. She is totally innocent about things in life. You don't get a second chance with Samantha. You know where you stand with Samantha.
Mother of Samantha, 21 years, BSL

They are happy in their life. I think they are better than hearing children. They, I don't know, they are more understanding or something.
Mother of Rosemary, 21 years, oral

INDEPENDENCE AND DEPENDENCE

We would like him to be away on his own, totally independent, and just come and visit us

Until now in this chapter, we have focused on the parents' perceptions of their sons and daughters. This is, of course, relevant to family relationships, particularly in respect of the young person's developing independence and the extent to which this is achieved, which we consider in this section. The age of the young people at the time of the interviews meant that they were at a period of transition from being a child to taking adult responsibilities in terms of relationships, living independently and becoming financially independent. In some respects we have seen that many of the young people had achieved these things, with an active social life and their own bank accounts, and some had left home.

However, there have also been indications of dependency and as the previous section has indicated some were seen as immature. It has emerged throughout the book that many parents were more involved in the lives of their sons and daughters than they would have been had they been hearing. Support was provided in finding work, job interviews and other interactions with the hearing world, including visits to doctors. Parents provided guidance in financial matters. They could have a small but significant responsibility for waking their son or daughter for work. They might also be involved in the social life of their son or daughter, through assisting with telephone conversations or passing on messages. For a small minority, the parents were involved in most aspects of day-to-day life. Most of these were necessary, because the hearing world is not adapted to the requirements of deaf people. Parents often stepped in because interpreters were not available or they were anxious about the services that were available. Other concerns would have been resolved by widespread provision of visual information systems or text telephones. Some parents did express the view that they had special concerns over their deaf sons and daughters compared with other members of the family.

I have always worried far more over Isabel than Victoria. I have always felt Victoria can take care, Victoria can cope. Victoria can do this and can do that. It never really felt that with Isabel. Isabel needs me. Now I had it said to me that I need Isabel more than Isabel needs me, and this may be perfectly true. This may be true, actually. I may be kidding myself that she needs me and it may be me that needs her. I don't know.
Mother of Isabel, 21 years, SSE

Put it like this. I am more worried about him than of his brother. If he goes out (the brother) and he's lost, he can ask or phone or something, but if Raj goes out and he's not back on time, I worry about how he's going to get in touch with me. In that sense maybe we are more protective, and we don't like to let them out of our sight, but it's not whites or Asians or anything like that, it's motherly instinct.
Mother of Raj, 23 years, BSL

Table 8.4. *Place of residence of young people*

	Number	%
Family home	52	63
Buying property	3	4
Renting house/flat/bedsit	13	16
Living with relatives/friends	6	7
College accommodation	5	6
Hostel/sheltered accommodation	3	4

Yet when they were asked if they saw their sons and daughters as independent or dependent, half (41, 50%) saw them as independent, less than a quarter (17, 21%) as dependent, and for the remaining 24 (29%), it varied. If we exclude the eight with limited language skills, who were all seen as dependent, only one in nine (9/74, 12%) were seen as still dependent.

A major step in achieving independence is leaving home, and Table 8.4 shows where the young people were living at the time of the parents' interviews. Just over one-third were living away from home, at least for part of the time. There was a clear ambivalence in some of the parents – although they wanted their sons and daughters to be independent, they also wanted to protect them. It may be the case that these families were particularly overprotective, though some did try to foster independence.

My husband said, 'Why do you bother?'. I said I think you bother because at the end of the day you want them out of your life, on their own two feet, locked away somewhere out of your life. At that distance you can cope with them.
Mother of Darren, 22 years, BSL

Some wanted their sons and daughters to leave home.

His behaviour is childish. He just wants all his own way. When we made him go, he didn't want to go. He was allowed a month to find somewhere to live.
Mother of James, 20 years, BSL

He won't leave home (laughs) we would like him to be away on his own, totally independent and just come and visit us like the rest of the family.
Mother of Darren 22 years, BSL

We are aware that the data we have presented cover a wide age range. We are also aware that, for some of these issues, the age span 18–24 years is wide. Things that are not surprising at 18 years may be at 24 years. We felt some readers might like to locate some of these findings with respect to a specific age, so we chose 20–21 years, the midpoint of which, 21, is the recent age of majority and still has some status.

Of the 40 in this group, 23 were seen as independent, ten as variable and seven as not independent. Most, (28/40, 70%) were living in the family home, one was buying a house, five were renting property, three were living with relatives and friends, two were at college and one was in a hostel. Other details are shown in Table 8.5.

As this chapter has outlined, because they live in a world which is almost exclusively geared to the needs of hearing people, many of the young people in our study were forced, in order to gain access to that world, to depend on their parents in a number of significant ways. However, the vast majority of them were developing independence.

FAMILY RELATIONSHIPS

Communication within the family

You are part of the family and I want you to be with us

In Chapter 2, we examined the nature of communication within the family. Many families experienced difficulty in communication, with implications, as we have seen, for the deaf young person. However, such factors could also influence family relationships. Communication within the family could be an effort, and other family members could feel excluded. Sometimes extra attention was given to managing social situations and often the mother took on significant responsibilities for communication.

Often, the stress came about, not through failure to communicate, but because families wanted to discuss things with each other.

Mother: We want to know such a lot, he wants to tell us a lot, but we find it tiring.
Father: Friday night when I came home from work, that was five o'clock and he had been talking to Pauline for, I presume, for an hour or so beforehand.
Mother: I said I felt tired.
Father: From five o'clock until probably half past six, when he went out, he probably never stopped.
Mother: But we can look back now and say, 'Don't we find it tiring?'

Table 8.5. *Measures of independence*
for 20- and 21-year-olds

Measure of independence	Number
Drive	
Yes	23
Learning	6
No	11
Take public transport alone	
Yes	38
No	2
Shop alone	
Yes	19
Sometimes	15
No	6
Visit the doctor's alone	
Yes	16
Sometimes	16
No	2
Manage finances	
Alone	20
With some help	16
No	4
Own bank account	
Yes	36
No	4

*But when he was here all the time, we didn't realise. But now we have
had a break from him, now we have to concentrate all the time. ( ) When
he does come home we realise how tired we get. It must have been like
that all the time.*
Parents of Phillip, 19 years, SSE

A number of parents made the point expressed in the previous quote, that
they became aware of the effort required after the son or daughter had left
home.

*There is always a strain. An atmosphere. And even now when he comes
home it is a strain. Unless it is me that worries, because he is always
telling me that I worry too much about him. But it is natural and you
have to make the effort of speaking to him, you see. When you have had
several days on your own or weeks on your own, then having to make a
conscious effort is quite noticeable. But we want him to come home as
much as possible.*
Mother of Robert, 22 years, BSL

It definitely puts a pressure on family life. It was a sense of relief when she left home. It was a relief to know that we could have people here without thinking about Christine feeling isolated. In a way, you feel guilty about it.
Mother of Christine, 21 years, SSE

There could also be a strain on general family relationships. This was an issue not just for the deaf young person but for other members of the family, and some siblings felt particularly resentful.

It makes a tremendous strain on the other children. Julie, the eldest, says, 'We never seem to have had a conversation, we're split into pieces'. And that still happens. It does annoy her, because I can't not answer him. When we're talking and he comes in and says, 'Mum', I immediately turn and answer him. Till this day she gets angry.
Mother of Darren, 22 years, BSL

Often, the family managed situations to make communication easier.

When we have groups of other people here, friends, or have gone to friends, it has always been a bit stressful, because you always have to be watching out for Janet, that she doesn't get left out and so on, knowing that she will not be too comfortable.
Mother of Janet, 22 years, oral

Sometimes specific plans were made.

For instance, the Christmas before last, we were going to my sister-in-law's and that meant there was going to be (list of 12 people) and he didn't think he would come at first and I was upset and I said, 'It is family, Colin, and you are part of the family and I want you to be with us. () So I contacted my sister-in-law and I explained what was happening and I said, 'Do you mind if we play "Give us a clue"?' () So my sister-in-law agreed and Colin said he would come, he would come for an hour and then he would go. But we got the games going and we eventually left at two o'clock in the morning and left them here!
Mother of Colin, 24 years, BSL

Often parents were aware of a responsibility in conveying information. While the young people pointed out how they missed things or were excluded from things, parents could perceive this as a responsibility.

I'll realise, 'Oh no, I haven't told her individually'. You just realise she's deaf again. She's not hearing – you have to tell her.
Mother of Fiona, 22 years, SSE

In many of these situations the major responsibility fell on the mother, as did the task of interpreting. With their 'special' degree of understanding, mothers often felt themselves to be informal interpreters even within the family.

> *I mean, the other day he said to Emma (sister), 'Where are you going this afternoon?' and she couldn't understand it. I had to shout down and tell her what he said, I shouted it down from upstairs. I could understand from upstairs what he was saying.*
> Mother of Gavin, 19 years, oral

> *He can't understand his Dad because every time his Dad asks him something he has to ask me what Dad says. I interpret for them.*
> Mother of Ivan, 21 years, BSL

We hope it is clear from these quotes that the parents did not resent or blame their sons and daughters for the situations described, and were more likely to feel guilt themselves. Often stress arose, not because families wanted to exclude the deaf member, but because they wanted them to be a part of the family in a full sense. And as we have already pointed out, it was not the deafness itself that was the issue, as families where all members are deaf communicate with ease, but the interface of the deaf and hearing worlds.

Husband–wife relationship

It brought us together, if anything. Though I can honestly see how it could break a marriage up

There are a number of reasons why one might expect the marriages of parents with deaf sons and daughters to be under particular pressure. Firstly, communication difficulties in the family would seem likely to lead to problems, and secondly, in the interviews, a significant number of parents talked of the stresses.

> *Oh yes, it has affected us in some ways. I know if Wayne is doing something wrong and we have told him off and we have had a real argument about it and we have argued together. But if Greg then starts telling me that it was a silly thing for him to do, it gets to me and then I want to stick up for him and then we start; that's the only time we start.*
> Mother of Wayne, 21 years, oral

Table 8.6. *Current state of marriage*

	Number	%
Marriage appears stable	36	46
Married, history of separations	4	5
Married, many rows reported	15	19
Total marriages intact	55	70
Death of one partner	4	5
Divorce	9	11
Separation	9	11
Death, but previous separation/divorce	2	3
Total divorce and separation	20	25

It reflects on the whole family, your marriage, because you are absolutely worn out. I look for support to Martin and Martin looks for support to me, and I mean my husband was brilliant, because when I would blow my stack he would keep cool. You know, where I would throw the papers in the air, Martin would keep very cool and calm. But nevertheless we were completely worn out at the end of the day.
Mother of Colin, 24 years, BSL

Yet these effects were not borne out in the findings, in terms of either the number of actual marriage breakdowns, or the parents feeling unhappy about marriage, nor was any consistency revealed about parental feelings when their son or daughter was a young child compared with when they were a young adult.

It is remarkably difficult to reach any clear-cut conclusions about the consequences for the marriage, as there are probably 82 different stories to be told with different family constitutions, different starting points and different attitudes to marriage. Also in the cause of marriage problems it is difficult to know what to attribute to the deafness, given that one-third of all marriages in the UK end in divorce. We have chosen to approach this topic in two ways, firstly by contrasting the state of the marriage now with that at the original interview, taking that as a baseline, even if at that time the marriage had broken up and a step-parent was already introduced. Our second perspective is to look at the accounts given of the marriage, and whether the parents themselves felt it had been enhanced or put under strain by the situation in which they found themselves.

Of the 82 interviewed, for two of the families there was no father at the time of the first interview and in a further one, there has been fostering since that time and relevant information is not available on the parents' marriage. Those three families are excluded from the analysis. Table 8.6

Table 8.7. *State of marriage now compared with feelings about marriage in earlier interview*

	Closer	Further apart	Same	Varies
Second interview				
Marriage appears stable	8	9	10	7
Married, history of separations	1	2	0	1
Married, many rows reported	2	2	5	4
Death of one partner	1	1	1	1
Divorce	1	1	2	4
Separation	1	1	0	1
Death, but previously separation/divorce	0	1	0	1
Total	14	17	20	21

shows the state of the marriage from information given at both parent and young people interviews. There seems to be no clear indication of a significant breakdown in the relationships beyond that of the general population. However, these data may be subject to certain limitations. It is possible, for example, that the losses from the sample contain a significantly higher incidence of marital breakdown than those retained.

The other interesting issue is whether marriage breakdown could be predicted from feelings about the marriage at the interview when the children were small. Of the 79 families, we have information from the earlier interview for 72. The results are given in Table 8.7. Although there may appear to be a slight tendency for those who said it varied early on to have the least stable marriages, none of the differences are statistically significant and show only chance variation.

Another perspective is to consider those 20 who at the later interviews were divorced or separated, or where a parent had died but there was a previous divorce or separation. In the interviews with this group of parents when the young person was a child, two had said the deafness brought them closer together, three that it drove them apart, eight that it varied, and four that it made no difference. Three did not answer the question at that time.

This confirmed our general impression in carrying out the interviews that although some parents did describe in detail pressures of the deafness on the marriage, it was not a critical influence for the marriage, which was affected to a greater extent by other factors. An alternative explanation could be that the effect of the deafness could be differential. It could result in the breakup of some marriages, but keep others together that might otherwise have broken down. Our own view, however, is that deafness was not usually the main determining factor.

Table 8.8. *Parents' perception of the effect of deafness on the marriage*

	Parent of deaf young child				
	No difference	Positive effect	Varies	Negative effect	Total
Parent of deaf young adult					
No difference	12	8	11	7	38
Positive effect	2	1	1	2	6
Varies	0	0	2	1	3
Negative effect	6	5	6	8	25
Total	20	14	20	18	72

We look now in more detail at consequences for the marital relationship in terms of the parents' perception of the situation. Breakdowns are only part of the story and may reveal little of the feelings about whether the deafness had affected the marriage. Table 8.8 shows the parents' perception of the effect of the deafness on the marriage at the two ages. This table is based on the 72 couples for whom the question was appropriate at both stages. Overall, there seems little consistency, positives have become negatives and vice versa. However, while twice as many parents reported that the deafness made no difference at the later stage than at the earlier stage, more were likely to report a negative than a positive effect. This may reflect a difference in the effect of deafness as the children grew up, but it could also indicate that the way in which people talked about their marriages in the early 1970s differed from that in the late 1980s.

This inconsistent pattern can be illustrated simply by taking as examples those marriages about which there were quotes in the first book. Divorce and separation can in no way be predicted from answers to the earlier question concerning feelings about marriage.

I think we argue more than we need do, don't we, because of the strain. It does put a strain on a marriage definitely.
Mother of Isabel, 6 years (DCF, p. 178)

No, it never pushed us apart. It brought us together, if anything. Though I can honestly see how it could break a marriage up.
Mother of Isabel, 21 years, SSE

I think whenever times of trouble crop up, that's when you find...I think I show signs of strain, it shows with my husband as well, and if I'd got a happy-go-lucky child that I'd got no worries over I'd be more relaxed with everyone. But you see I get short tempered, and then the strain shows with his family...
Mother of Jane, 4 years (DCF, p. 178)

I can't stand the strain of it, either. But then what happens was, with this house going wrong, everything had rusted up, my husband and I weren't getting on. So it would have come to that, you can't live together where someone's under constant strain, something has got to give.
Mother of Jane, 20 years, oral

Yet in one family that reported deafness bringing them closer together, the marriage has ended in divorce.

I don't know whether it's Samantha, but I think we're more in love now than ever we were. I don't know whether love grows in marriage. You see, you don't really know, because you don't compare anybody else's marriage to your own, do you? I mean, it's not driven us apart, I'll give it that.
Mother of Samantha, 4 years (DCF, p. 180)

One possibility is that having a deaf son or daughter does change the marriage, but not in the same way or in a negative way for all couples, so some it drives apart and some it brings closer together. Another interpretation could be that it affects marriages by exaggerating the general position, bringing those who were close, closer, and driving those who were stressed, further apart.

I just think it makes your marriage hard if you have not got a particularly good marriage. I think it is just that bit that forces you. It definitely puts a strain on your marriage and if you have got a rocky one that is just it. Because you seem to have to spend that much more time than you would.
Mother of Bridget, 22 years, BSL

I know we were close enough together anyway, but having a deaf kid you close ranks. () I mean, we can't really bicker between ourselves because we have got enough on our plate.
Father of Sharon, 21 years, BSL

The deaf young people, as other young people, were often very opposed to any marriage breakup.

Mother: It was when me and her Dad split up.
Interviewer: How did she take that?
Mother: Not very well, she wanted me to have her Dad back.
Interviewer: Did she?
Mother: Yes, well her Dad were bribing her, you know what I mean. She keeps saying, 'Why don't you want my Dad to come back?' and how

can you explain as how you don't. She kept on saying, 'Why?' That were difficult, that. And when I started going out with somebody she didn't like him. That caused a lot of trouble. Mind you, she's not liked any of them.
Mother of Bridget, 22 years, BSL

This was confirmed in the interviews with the young people who were usually depressed at any tension in the marriage and particularly if the marriage broke down, whatever the reasons.

Father left. I love my father, but at the same time I think he is cruel, the way he used to hit my mother. When they split up I was depressed and sad.
Bobby, 20 years, SSE

I was very angry when they split up. I am happy living with my father, but he wants my Mum back and so do I.
Melanie, 18 years, BSL

Sibling relationships

It has got to be a very special person who would not feel some resentment

Little is known in general about sibling relationships. A recent study reiterating this, also said that there is little consistency in the overall pattern, although critical events tend to exaggerate the existing state of the relationship (Dunn & Kendrick, 1982). The variety of sibling relationships can be as varied, or more so, than marital ones. Siblings can be older or younger to varying degrees, brothers or sisters, deaf or not deaf.

Relationships can also vary within one family, as the following quote shows:

They understand him, no problem. Andrew can use sign language because he's learnt it. His eldest sister, he doesn't like very much. She's always resented him, he was taken ill the day she started school. She makes an effort when she feels like it but he knows its an effort. His youngest sister, he likes her. She's very kind, patient, and laughs at him but always treats him as an equal. His other sister doesn't, she tends to talk down to him.
Mother of Darren, 22 years, BSL

However, there were issues raised about siblings and rather than try to construct an overall picture we have tried to draw out some of the main themes. Of the 82 young people for whom the parents were interviewed, 79 had siblings. Of these, three had siblings who were much younger than themselves, so it has not been appropriate to include them in all the analyses. Twelve of the young people had deaf brothers or sisters, and four of them had siblings with other disabilities (one was blind, one had cerebral palsy, one had learning difficulties and one had acquired speech disabilities as a consequence of a road accident).

Overall, the relationship with the siblings was described in positive terms by the parents, with 45 (57%) seen as having a good relationship, 23 (29%) having a good relationship with some siblings but not with others, four (5%) being indifferent to their siblings and only in seven instances (9%) was the relationship actually seen as negative. The young people too felt the relationships to be generally positive, with 23 (42%) describing themselves as getting on very well with their siblings, 19 (35%) quite well, 11 (20%) differentiating between siblings and only two (4%) saying they did not get on well at all. A direct comparison is not made between these, as the basis for the parents' and young people's judgment was different. The parents judged the mutual relationship between two people, whereas the young people described how well they themselves got on with their siblings.

Despite this generally positive picture, in the interviews there emerged a number of causes for concern, particularly on the part of the parents. One of these was the need to spend more time with the deaf child and the consequences of this.

> *They don't feel it themselves. When he was at boarding school they used to pray for the weekend to go, because he was such a nuisance.*
> *Mother of James, 20 years, BSL*

And some parents felt that resentment was inevitable.

> *I think it would be very difficult for (sister) to admit that, but in all honesty it has got to be a very special person who would not feel some sort of resentment, because a deaf person alters the lives of everyone in a home. It is a big big disturbance in everything you do.*
> *Mother of Colin, 24 years, BSL*

In Chapter 3, it was suggested that boarding school could be very disruptive to family relationships. Nicky was sent to boarding school when she was three, a few months before her sister Helen was born. At first it was policy only to allow them home once every two weeks. At the time Nicky's mother said:

This is a real problem, because Nicky's away for a fortnight, home for a weekend, away for a fortnight, home for a weekend. Well, for the fortnight, Helen has me every time she wants me, because there is no one else wanting me, and then for the weekends Nicky needs me so much, because she has been away, and Helen thinks, naturally, that she's the one, that whenever she cries she can come to me, and they won't be nursed together, they won't be loved together, and I try to make up to Nicky for what she's missed by being away and I try not to let Helen feel she's been pushed out, but I'm sure she does feel it, because often when Nicky's home she wakes up more at nights, and we sit together at night, Helen and I and she has ten minutes' cuddle. I don't think we can do anything about it, except trying to avoid having them both upset at the same time.
Mother of Nicky, 4 years (DCF, p. 181)

Not surprisingly, throughout their lives there had been jealousy between them which their mother described at the interview. She says of their relationship now:

There is a certain amount of tension between Nicky and Helen. () They live separate lives under the same roof. They care about each other but they wouldn't choose to go out with each other.
Mother of Nicky, 21 years, SSE

This mother, too, in the later interview described how boarding school had been an influential factor in the relationship between the two sisters. Teresa has boarded since she was seven years.

(About boarding school from 14 years) She didn't want to go back at all when she came home. Boring all the while. You tend to pamper her a little when she was at home. She thought she was missing out on things while she was away at school, her sister would be getting more than she was. There is a lot of jealousy between her and her sister.
Mother of Teresa, 22 years, BSL

However, although boarding school was a significant factor in a number of situations, and seen as the cause, in fact there was more jealousy between siblings and deaf young people who attended other settings, according to the parents' perception, as is seen in Table 8.9. Whereas two-thirds of those attending schools for the deaf had positive relationships with their siblings, only half of those in PHUs or mainstream settings did. However, while the difficulty for those who went to boarding school is usually attributed to the effect of boarding, in the other situations, the educational setting was not mentioned in the context of sibling conflict.

Table 8.9. *Relationship between siblings and the type of school attended*

Schooling	Relationship between siblings	
	Positive	Negative, indifferent or mixed
Mainstream	4	6
Deaf (boarding)	20	11
Deaf (non-boarding)	8	4
Partially Hearing Unit	12	11

Sometimes, relationships between siblings were close and positive. In a number of instances it seemed to us that this was in situations where, when the children were young, the mother had tried to discuss feelings with the hearing sibling.

> *I don't think she really understands. It's only recently she's said to me, 'I wish Gary wasn't deaf and I say, 'I do as well, Sarah, and we have to try and help him in this way' and this is it. Sarah's very sensitive, but I don't think she understands fully. We try and include her in everything. We always had...*
> *Mother of Gary, 3 years (DCF, p. 182)*

> *Yes, I think so. Not all the time, but I think sometimes I'm inclined to, I think. Janet knows like, Sharon has to have more attention. We've explained to her, you know that she has to have more attention because she can't hear and Janet's very good with her.*
> *Mother of Sharon, 4 years old (DCF, p. 181).*

> *Father: I mean Janet, when she was living at home she was close to her anyway.*
> *Mother: Very, very close. Even now she is married, even Peter her husband, he is absolutely fantastic. He has never walked in here and ignored her and neither has any of her family.*
> *Father: It was funny, really, the night of the wedding. It got to about midnight, and she sat down and cried, Sharon did, didn't she?*
> *Mother: I went to her and said, 'What is the matter?' () and Sharon cried, 'He's taken you away from me' and that is all she said, and Peter said to her ()*
> *Father: 'I haven't taken her away, you've gained me!' he said.*
> *Parents of Sharon, 21 years, BSL*

We also asked whether there was any feeling in the family on the part of the brothers and sisters of the deaf young person of future responsibility for them. Of the 74 for whom this question was appropriate (excluding those with no siblings and five more instances where the sibling would be unable to take responsibility), 46 (62%) were described as having some sense of future responsibility, though in the majority of cases this was to keep in touch or to keep an eye on things and only four were seen as expecting to provide a home for their deaf brother or sister. Twenty-five (34%) felt no responsibility and in three instances the parents did not feel they knew.

Occasionally, the impact of the young person's deafness was not on the sibling relationship, but feelings about future children.

> *Both her and her husband have said that if they bring a handicapped child into the world, if they know it is handicapped before birth, they will have it terminated. If it is born handicapped they are going to put it up for adoption. Amanda would not be able to take it. They have said this. She said, 'I have had 18 years, Mum, and I don't want a lifetime with the handicapped'. She wouldn't cope, it's not an easy decision to make but she has said it.*
> *Mother of Melanie, 18 years, BSL*

Other family members

They know she's favourite

As we have seen in Chapter 3, it was a cause for sadness among some of the young people that their communication with members of the extended family was not as they felt it should be. Often grandparents were mentioned, and they too sometimes found the relationship different.

> *My mother has the most difficulty with him. She's never at ease with Darren.*
> *Mother of Darren, 22 years, BSL*

More often, though, the problem was the reverse. Rather than grandparents being unfriendly or rejecting to their deaf grandsons and granddaughters they could favour them to the detriment of brothers and sisters. In one family a substantial sum of money was left to the deaf grandson with nothing to his sister, creating a problem for the parents.

In another instance, the daughter left home to live with the grandmother.

> *The first grandchild. She spoilt her rotten. When she first left school she went to live with her grandmother.*
> *Interviewer: Why was that?*
> *Well, she couldn't do as she liked with me, and she would go up there you see, and her Grandma used to sympathise with her.*

Later in the interview the mother described how her daughter had exploited the grandmother.

> But she has had no end of money off her grandmother, though – taken money off her. Took it out of her purse and all sorts.
> Interviewer: Really, and her grandmother didn't mind.
> Her Grandma daren't say nothing. () She went to people's houses and said Grandma wants to borrow £5. No end of people had come and asked for it. I said, 'It's their fault for giving it to her'. She is very crafty in that. () And Grandma paid up what she had. I wouldn't have done it.
> Mother of Bridget, 22 years, BSL

This favouritism had resulted in some jealousy among the siblings.

> They know she's favourite. They say, 'Grandma always gives it her'.
> Interviewer: Do they resent it?
> They do a bit.
> Mother of Bridget, 22 years, BSL

In the following situation the grandma, through her attitude, affected the whole family.

> Grandma, Martin's mother, absolutely idolised him in a way that was insensitive, and she caused a lot of resentments between Colin and Pauline, because she idolised Colin and he could have the earth, he could have anything he wanted and Pauline got nothing.
> Interviewer: Why do you think that was?
> It was because he was a boy and because he was handicapped. () She bought Colin a television and it was his and Pauline was not to watch it. So we had big family arguments. It was worse, because Colin knew the television was his and we wouldn't allow it in the house. And she thought I was a cruel mother, and this all adds to the problems between husband and wife, because she thought I was a cruel mother in the way I tried to make Colin independent, the way I made him work, listening to sounds and everything. I mean I wasn't cruel, but she thought I should have done everything for him, I shouldn't have let him make any effort. And she would have wrapped him in cotton wool, that's all she wanted to do.
> Mother of Colin, 24 years, BSL

Despite the dramatic nature of some of these situations and the links made with deafness, it was very difficult to say whether or not there was a major effect.

THE EFFECT ON THE PARENTS' LIFE

As we reported in the last chapter, when we asked the young people if their deafness had affected their family they found it a difficult question to answer. Of the 41 who could answer, 25 (61%) saw negative consequences, although in many instances these were in the past rather than contemporaneous. When we asked the parents about pressures on the family, 41 (50%) said there were considerable pressures and 28 (34%) that there were slight pressures. The responses did not show a relationship with the preferred language of the young person.

We asked more specific questions about social life, work and health to see how the pressures were experienced in the different areas. At the time of the interview, only 17 (17/81, 21%) felt their social life to be affected and only four (5%) of these to any considerable extent. The effects seem to have been greater in the past, with 29 (29/80, 36%) describing consequences for their social life and 15 (19%) of these being considerable. If we compare these results with those of the first interview, we find little consistency with accounts of social life then, although the measures are not directly comparable. However, there is a consistency if we compare the mother's perception of whether the deafness affected her life, in general, at the first interview, with the later effect on social life. All those reporting a considerable effect later, had earlier reported that the deafness had changed their lives and three-quarters (10/13) of those with a slight effect now had reported an effect then.

Some parents, however, rather than describing a negative effect, suggested that it had improved their social life.

> *I think we've got to know a lot of people than we would have done otherwise. I think we've been to places we wouldn't have been. I think because of the deafness, ( ) we've organised things that we'd never have done, we've been to places we'd never have gone to, we've done things we'd never have done.*
> Mother of Veronica, 21 years, SSE

Very few of the families reported a consequence for their work or careers. Where there was an effect, in nine instances it was for the father and in six for the mother. Effects on the father did not relate to any effects reported at the earlier interview but all eight of the mothers who said their work had been affected had earlier said that the deafness had made a significant difference to their lives.

The mothers' health was a concern at the first interview, when 7% were in poor health, 28% had some health problems and 4% felt themselves to be run down. At this later interview about one in ten (10/82, 12%) were experiencing poor health and one-third (26/82, 32%) moderate health problems. This increase is probably due to age factors as much as anything else. At the later interview we asked to what extent the problems could be attributed to the deafness and a majority, seven of those with considerable problems and 17 with moderate problems, saw this as a factor. However, health problems at the early interview were not a predictor of later health problems.

A focus on problems creates a negative perspective, so it is important to note that overall problems occurred for the minority of families, 81% experienced no problems with work, 56% no health problems, and 79% no problems with social life. Such as there were, were not predicted by any specific features of their early life. However, there was an overall tendency for those who saw the deafness as affecting their lives in a general sense at the first interview, to have more problems later on. It is an area of dispute, however, whether the problems were in excess of those that might be described by parents of hearing young people.

COMING TO TERMS WITH DEAFNESS

I was just sheer relieved to know it wasn't me going mad

Maybe, however, the most important consequence for the parents was coming to terms with deafness, and making sense of their child's deafness in the context of their own lives. The time of diagnosis was a critical time, and the events surrounding diagnosis were remembered with dramatic clarity by the vast majority of the families. It was remarkable that the words used to describe the events around diagnosis were often very similar at the two interviews, which were 17 or 18 years apart. There are very many examples that we could have chosen, but we include only a few here. The first is in response to a question about how they found out their child was deaf.

> *Well it were the lady next door that told me. She dropped the coal bucket on the hearth, when he was a baby this was, about eight month old, and she says he never flinched. And so we took him to the doctor's.*
> Mother of Brian, 5 years old

> *Well, it were the neighbour next door that told me. She dropped the coal bucket and he was lying on the settee and he never flinched. She got*

some bells and rang them at the side of him and he never gave no response. So I took him to the doctor's and she sent me down to the Children's Hospital at Nottingham. So he was going there, say from eight months, yes, until I think he was over two.
Mother of Brian, 22 years old, LLS

A further question asked what the doctor had actually said to them at the time.

Your child is sort of deaf, and not just a little. We must get something done.
Mother of Tom, 4 years old

He was very very quiet and made the picture look so black. 'Your child is deaf and very severely deaf and we must get something done right away and why was this not brought to my notice earlier?'
Mother of Tom, 20 years old, BSL

The mothers were also asked how they felt at the time.

I was just sheer relieved to know it wasn't me going mad, at first. So many people had stood in my path and said, 'You're whittling, you're worrying – there's nothing wrong with her, she'll talk when she's ready'. I thought if it went on much longer at home and that child was supposed to be normal, I'd go off me rocker. So really it wasn't so much finding fault with anybody, or how it had been handled, it was just a relief to think that at long last we did know there was something wrong, and what it was, and could tackle it.
Mother of Jane, 4 years old

It's so difficult to remember what it was like at the time. I think, when you feel there is something wrong all along and you couldn't put your finger on it, knowing something is a relief in a way, it takes the worry out of it, and the wondering whether you were imagining it or going mad or wondering, is it this, is it that. When somebody says – it's that, it's a big relief.
Mother of Jane, 20 years old, oral

The uniqueness of the event seems to have made an indelible impression, such that often the very words used ('relief'), or the emotions described ('going mad') are identical. It may be a situation that relates to people's memories of where they were when particular traumatic events are made public, such as when the news of Kennedy's assassination became known.

In the report of the first study, there is a chapter which is concerned with coming to terms with deafness. It was written as if it were a task to be accomplished. However, the later interviews have made it apparent to us that this is an ongoing process. Coming to terms with a deaf baby is very different from coming to terms with a deaf teenager, a deaf young person, a deaf adult. Parents who were very accepting of a deaf baby were often shocked to find how ill prepared they were when the baby became a deaf school child, or when careers were discussed in terms of careers for deaf people, or when their sons' and daughters' lives were spent mostly with other deaf people and most of their friends were deaf.

Not only did the parents have to address their own feelings about deafness, but they often had to explain aspects of the deafness to their sons and daughters, including why they were deaf or that they would always be deaf. The parents had to deal with any unhappiness experienced by the young people, and address their concerns about whether or not they would become hearing.

I can remember, it brought tears to my eyes. She said, 'When I grow up and I can hear', she thought she would hear when she grew up. She was younger than ten years of age when she said this. It was awful having to tell her she'd never hear.
Mother of Zoe, 19 years, BSL

Father: Because when he was a kid he used to say, 'When I grow up and I can hear properly' didn't he?
Mother: 'When I grow up and I can hear properly I won't wear those.'
Father: I think he only thought it was really because he was a kid, you know.
Parents of Wayne, 21 years, oral

I had always hoped there would be an operation

In the last chapter we saw how the majority of the deaf young people saw their deafness as an integral part of themselves; they could not conceive of life in any other way. For the hearing parents, though, it was different. None of them had expected to have a deaf child, and most of them still occasionally thought about the hearing child that might have been. Few of them had any contact with deaf people before their own child was born, and the birth of their deaf child meant that family life was very different for them from the way they had expected it to be. It has to be said that none of the hearing parents had wanted their child to be deaf and none of them came to regard it as a blessing, in the way that has been suggested by a member of the Deaf community (Oliver, 1989). This does not detract in any way from the positive relationship that existed between most of the parents and their sons and daughters and the genuine love and affection the parents felt.

I know it sounds stupid, but I still don't accept 100% that he is going to be deaf – you still feel at the back of your mind (it sounds crazy, doesn't it?) that one day the miracle is going to happen and one day he is going to hear. I know now he is much more comfortable in a deaf world and all I want is for him to be happy anyway – I want him to have what makes him happiest.
Mother of Colin, 24 years, BSL

I have always hoped that there will be an operation but whether I am...I don't know. Its complicated. It is the most complicated organ in the body. And how minute this cochlea is, which is really where Isabel and a lot of kids' damage actually is. It is going to be...
Mother of Isabel, 21 years, SSE

I asked if I could have her ears X-rayed again. They said it wasn't worth it. Probably it would have been a waste, but at least I could see what I was looking at, and thinking, 'Well, there can't be anything done'. At least when you can't see it you keep hoping. If I thought tomorrow they said in Australia they would knit nerves on ears and she could have it done, I would take her.
Father of Shirley, 22 years, SSE

One-third (27, 33%) of the parents said they had sought a cure for the deafness. Five had visited Lourdes, two had looked into alternative medicine. Cochlear implants were seen as having the greatest potential and 23 families had enquired about these.

You feel cheated in a lot of ways

Within the Deaf community there is much discussion of Deaf culture, and the need for deaf people from hearing families to have access to this. It can be forgotten, though, that hearing parents, too, have a culture they expected and wanted to share with their deaf sons and daughters.

When they are deaf there is no God, no Jesus, no bedtime stories, no fairy stories, just nothing.
Mother of Robert, 22 years, BSL

She was saying to me, 'You know, I have never known a nursery rhyme'. And I said, 'Janet, I must have told you nursery rhymes!' She said, 'You

haven't, because I don't know them and I feel a fool now when I don't know them'. I said, 'I must have done' and she said, 'You can't have done'. I said, 'What must have happened was I was so busy telling you other things that I missed out on that'. I can't imagine that I would have done, but then perhaps I was so busy saying, 'This is a table' that I missed out on it.
Mother of Janet, 22 years, oral

You feel, actually, with young deaf children, cheated in a lot of ways, because they do not learn nursery rhymes. I mean, Carol has never taken to tunes or anything like that, has she? You know how you sing little songs to them and that () you feel as if you have been done out of something.
Mother of Carol, 23 years, oral

There is so much unhappiness and heartache. It is the terrible heartache of living among normal hearing people and seeing your son who is the misfit wanting to be part of it, and it is the realisation, you know, just how much he is going to miss out of life. It makes you very very unhappy.
Mother of Colin, 24 years, BSL

The cultural issues were magnified for families from the minority ethnic groups, where their family culture and often their home language was different from that of the dominant society. Most of them described their sons and daughters as being integrated with the local Deaf community but not with their family community, despite the fact that they would be welcome there. For most of the families, spending time with other members of their community was important – there were many family celebrations, parties and festivals. Sometimes the young people were persuaded to go to them, but often it was accepted that as they became older they preferred to spend the time with their deaf friends.

It's sad. He's lost some things. If there is a wedding or something, he won't come. He says he hasn't got any friends there, and I wouldn't want to force him, no.
Mother of Ritesh, 24 years, BSL

There is a language barrier, because the signing is in English, and not all Asian families speak English, and that is very difficult. There is no reason for them to get together with the Asian group. They want to be with their own group, exchange ideas, have a meeting, have a party. At least they are there for each other to rely on.
Father of Raj, 23 years, BSL

This last quote raises an important issue, for although, for most of the particular families we talked to, the young people had attended a school for the deaf and were in a city with a strong Asian Deaf Club, this would not be the same for many young people from minority ethnic communities.

One family felt that they would have been better able to cope with the deafness had they been living in India, as, despite there being a significant Asian community where they lived, there were not enough people to meet their son's needs.

Being Asian is a problem, because we have not many population here. If I was in India it would be different again. I could show him many things. But because we are here and because we are Asian that is a problem. () This is a different country and we are not the original people.
Father of Anil, 23 years, BSL

GREATER UNDERSTANDING

I think it has made me a better person

We feel the parents in this study were confronted with a number of decisions that were different in quality and degree from those faced by hearing parents. Some felt this had increased their understanding of a number of issues and while they were never asked explicitly to comment on this, a number did so in response to a question about whether their family life would have been different if their son or daughter had not been deaf.

I think it's made us all more tolerant of other people and particularly of other people with a handicap.
Mother of Josie, 24 years, BSL

In some ways it has been better, because it has made me aware, not just of the deafness disability, but of other disabilities, and it has made me think about other people's problems. It's certainly made me control my temper.
Mother of Nicky, 21 years, SSE

In some ways, richer. I've learnt a lot about children. Wouldn't have missed it for anything really. When she was about nine, she asked why she was deaf. Did we want a deaf daughter? It must have been a good enough answer, because she did not come back with it.
Mother of Tina, 18 years, oral

I wouldn't have developed as I have developed, I am sure. It'd made me into a stronger and more determined person. I think it makes you more tolerant of other disabilities.
Mother of Zoe, 19 years, BSL

I think by nature I'm very intolerant. I don't like slowness of mind or body. I like when I talk to people I want a real answer. I'm intolerant and it's taught me not to be.
Mother of Veronica, 21 years, SSE

I think it has made me a better person.
Mother of Gary, 20 years, oral

It does widen your life, definitely, because it makes you think a lot more about other handicaps. You watch a programme on television and you think, 'Gosh, I didn't realise that!' I mean when you first get involved in this business of bringing up a deaf child you tend to go stomping round saying, 'People don't understand, nobody considers what it is like' but of course they don't, because you wouldn't have done it yourself.
Mother of Carol, 23 years, oral

CHAPTER NINE

Reflections

In this chapter we take the opportunity to reflect upon the findings presented in this book and try to draw some of the central themes together. We also review the relationship between the parent's and young person's perspective and examine some of the changes in parental perspective over time. We discuss the implications of the findings and look to the future for the deaf young people and their families.

In doing this, we cannot be comprehensive, but only selective. The implications are those we have chosen to draw from the research, and other people may see other issues as more significant. Yet others, from their reading of the same evidence, may draw different conclusions from those that we suggest.

THEMES AND ISSUES

Language and communication

A pervasive theme of this book has been language and communication. This has been expressed in a number of ways and at several levels. A basic issue has been the linguistic competence of the young people, regardless of the language they used. In some situations, the ability to access spoken language was also significant. Beyond this, the familiarity of the young people with conversations, reflecting on their own experience and describing their own point of view has been discussed. All these concerns have consequences for the young people and for family life.

A proportion of the young people were linguistically competent and gave careful and thoughtful answers to the interview. Of the 61 young people interviewed, nearly one-third (19, 31%) scored highly on a scale measuring the ability to give complex answers, and nearly one-fifth (11, 18%) scored highly on a scale measuring the ability to understand complex questions. Most (36, 59%) could understand the straightforward questions measured by the scale. For some, though, the interview was more difficult. From the 82 families interviewed, 14 (17%) of the young people could not be interviewed in a way that allowed for their responses to be used in the quantitative analysis. This is considered in Chapter 1 and further discussed in Chapter 8. Even those young people who did participate, were not always able to answer all of the questions or sense could not always be made of their responses. This is apparent from the presentation of data throughout the book, where virtually all analyses of young people's responses include a category for the number not answering. Comprehension of questions and the ability to give complex responses could not be taken for granted. Overall, a pessimistic picture of the linguistic abilities of a substantial proportion of the young deaf people has emerged. We were further struck by the fact that many had rarely had experience of answering questions about themselves. While sometimes we were restricted in the interviews by limitations in their language ability, at other times it was their lack of experience of thinking about, and reflecting upon, issues raised in the interviews.

Within some families good communication was established, while for others it was more difficult. For virtually all families language and communication were an issue. Many parents regretted that they could not have the same ease of communication with their deaf sons and daughters that they did with those who were hearing. Easy communication not only has a role in facilitating the practicalities of day-to-day life, but is intrinsic to the development of self esteem and identity. Many writers on adolescence stress the importance of good family communication for such development and the following quote is typical:

> *Communication is a crucial aspect of family life, affecting the quality of the relationship between the parents and the healthy functioning of both individual family members and the family as a whole. In particular, supportive communication in the family encourages the development of more positive identities among adolescents and higher levels of social and coping skills.*
>
> *Noller & Callan (1991)*

If ease of communication could not be taken for granted in the family, it could inhibit the young deaf person's ability to give accounts of themselves, their feelings, hopes and aspirations. It could limit discussions on issues around growing up. It could also mean the young deaf person was less well informed about family events and less participating in family decisions and thus less able to feel a full member of the family, all of which could have consequences for the emergent identity and self esteem of the young person. Not only could this have consequences for the young person, but other family members could feel they had additional responsibilities. Often the mother or another person acted as interpreter within the family. Conversation at family events was sometimes 'managed' so that the young deaf person could be involved. Often parents saw themselves as having a particular responsibility to keep the young deaf person informed, both within particular situations, and about family life in general.

We have already pointed out that difficulties in communication are not an inevitable consequence of deafness and have described how communication in families where all parents and young people are deaf can be taken for granted in the same way as it is in hearing families. However, the issue is at the interface of the deaf and hearing worlds. The discussion of signing throughout the book may seem simply to lead to the conclusion that all that is necessary is for families to learn to sign. Certainly most families felt that they should have had that opportunity, and signing should have been offered to them. If family members did learn to sign, regardless of the level of competence achieved, this was almost invariably viewed by the deaf young person in a positive way, as an acceptance of their deafness, with consequences for their self esteem. However, the use of signing is itself a complex option and is discussed later in the chapter.

Difficulties in language and communication had an impact on the lives of the young people in the outside hearing world. For the young people it could mean that day-to-day interactions that hearing people take for granted could be a strain. Even when young people felt at ease with their families, in the outside hearing world they could be more disadvantaged. Those for whom sign language was their preferred language were dependent on the ability of others to sign, or the use of interpreters, an expensive and rare resource. Those who relied on lip reading and listening could find conversations in groups a strain.

As the father of Carol pointed out:

> *But it makes you wonder, too, what she is thinking about things. You don't really know. From the moment she puts her foot into the office in the morning, is she feeling, 'Gosh, now I've got to start' and 'Have I got to watch out for who is talking and the direction the sound is coming from and what they are saying if I want to join in?' I mean they are bantering, they have a banter in the office. 'I have got to watch out if I am to be included, otherwise they can chat away and it is so much fresh*

*air'. Babble goes over the top. With everything, in order to be part of it,
she had got to make the effort.*
Father of Carol, 23 years, oral

Despite their best efforts, conversation for the young deaf person could be
trying to make sense based on little information.

*If she is in a conversation she will not pick the whole of the conversation
up, she will take little bits out and she roughly understands what you
were talking about.*
Father of Sharon, 21 years, BSL

Not only did this affect the lives of young people but it had sometimes
resulted in the development of strategies to make it appear that they were
understanding.

*The only thing I can remember being really shaken about was when she
was at the comprehensive – one afternoon instead of their English
lesson they took them into the theatre to watch a rehearsal of a play and
Carol came home and said they had been to see this play and 'It was very
good, I enjoyed it very much, it was funny'. And I said, 'Well, could you
hear? Could you hear the jokes?' She said, 'Oh no, I couldn't hear it, I
just laughed when everybody else did'. And that really set me back on
my heels, that. I thought what a dreadful thing to have to admit, and she
didn't seem to think there was anything wrong about it at all. I thought
it was terribly sad. It really upset me very badly, that.*
Mother of Carol, 23 years, oral

This quote resonates with that of the young man quoted in Chapter 2 who
said that he wanted to laugh at the same time as the others. It also
reinforces the notion mentioned above and elsewhere in the literature that
the appearance of being part of the social situation can be more important
than actually understanding what is going on. Nodding, smiling, saying
'yes' or 'no' are features of deaf children's behaviour at school that have
been noted in the literature (Gregory & Bishop, 1991; Lynas, 1986). We
ourselves were also aware in the interview that the desire to please us was
often more important to the young people than understanding the
questions and answering them fully. Often there were nods and smiles and
vague responses to questions that were not fully understood.

Access to information

Ease of language and communication has a clear and immediate significance for relationships and for day-to-day life. However, there was

another consequence of deafness for the young people that seemed to us of equal significance, but that has not always been given the same degree of attention. Although this issue has not been discussed as a specific section in this book, access to information has emerged over and over again as a significant issue for deaf people. The ability to access incidental information, overhear or oversee conversations, or note something in passing, should never be underestimated. One of the things that has struck us throughout the research is the lack of information available to the deaf person in terms of expectations, appropriateness of behaviour, understanding of how various systems function. This has an impact on their lives and that of their families who take a greater role than they might otherwise in the young person's life. Although less tangible, it seems to us that the impact of this is as significant as language and communication.

Limited access to conversation and the spoken word had major consequences for the young person's developing understanding of the world. While some knowledge can be acquired directly by being told, or from formal tuition, for hearing people most of their understanding of the world – what is happening, how things work – is acquired indirectly through casual conversation, through overhearing, or through television or radio, even when attention is only partial.

> *You realise that hearing people pick up a lot of worldly things where deaf people they have got to be told it, and sometimes you don't realise the things they accept that you know they don't know.*
> Mother of Phillip, 19 years, SSE

In very many places in the book it has emerged that the young people have been denied full participation in their world through lack of knowledge. In terms of understanding about career choice, prospects and possibilities at work, and managing financial affairs, often it was not language that was the issue, but the lack of access to information. This could apply to knowledge of local and world events.

> *We don't have problems understanding what she's saying. We sometimes have problems understanding what she **means** because she is confused in her ideas and conceptions. It's very difficult explaining things like local government. I mean, she's interested in the news and what's happening in the world, but it is difficult to explain the wider implications of current affairs to her. She doesn't know the background of how the government works.*
> Mother of Fiona, 22 years, SSE

It may be tempting in this instance to say that most young people do not understand how the government works anyway. However, the fact that this mother chose to mention it, meant it violated her own expectations of what her daughter should know and is thus significant.

Parents themselves, who knew the young people well, were often taken aback by gaps in their knowledge. A number of anecdotes from the interviews may make the point more vividly. One mother recounted how her daughter, who was learning to drive, had never been told, and thus did not realise, that learner drivers are only allowed to drive when accompanied by another driver.

> *She has been learning. And there is a funny story to this, because one day when Peter (husband) went out in his car and I came home, she said, 'Do you know Mum, I don't like my Dad's car, it's too big, but yours is lovely'. And I said, 'What do you mean, lovely?' And she said, 'I took your car out for a drive', and I said, 'When?' And she said, 'This afternoon. And I said, 'Melanie, you're only a learner. How did you get it off the drive?' She said, 'I have had my lessons, I put it into reverse with no problems'. I said, 'Did you put the L-plates on?' 'No.' 'Nobody with you? Who saw you?'() I said, 'You do realise you are not allowed to drive a car without a driver being with you'. 'My driving instructor said perhaps I could go out and practice in your car.' I said, 'Do you realise that you haven't got insurance and you haven't got L-plates?' 'Oh' she said, 'nobody told me'.*
> *Mother of Melanie, 18 years, BSL*

Two parents recounted stories involving misunderstandings about money.

> *There was one time he just walked into a shop in the village and just walked out again with it. He didn't seem to understand he had to pay for things. He was about 12, I think, although he didn't go for things a lot on his own.*
> *Mother of Ivan, 21 years, BSL*

Robert's mother told how when he was nine or ten he had been found giving out large sums of money at school, which he had taken from his father's shop.

> *You feel so terribly guilty that you have not explained money and what it was for. You don't realise that you have to do it! Because he didn't know what all this money was for and where it was from. It was from the shop. He had never seen it before in his life at school and it didn't mean anything. He just saw his father counting out money ready to bank and he obviously didn't know where it came from, because*

nobody explained to him. You see the everyday course of life, living, is
completely foreign to him, because he can't hear.
Mother of Robert, 22 years, BSL

Another mother told a story where it was not lack of information that was
the issue, but information that had been misunderstood, where her
daughter had not been fully able to discuss things that had been described
to her.

I can think of something I must tell you. A midwife on the doorstep.
'We've had a cry for help, one of your daughters is pregnant.' (laughs)
Well, what had happened, this was when she worked on YTS. She will
not accept that babies have to have blood tests. She gets very upset
about things like that. For some time she'd been on to us and to
everybody, she says how cruel it is to prick a baby! Even smacking it to
make it cry when it's born, that's cruel. We tried our best to get her to
understand it's in the baby's best interests and the baby would not
remember it. () She'd written all over the country. It was amazing. ()
She'd sent the letter and bought all the stamps, she didn't get any replies
soon enough so she'd sent another letter.
Interviewer: What did the letter say?
She told them off, didn't they know it hurt the baby, how cruel it was.
Mother of Fiona, 22 years, SSE

The following mother described how her son thought the world had
become coloured at a particular point in time as photographs and
television pictures of the past were always black and white.

Harry came home one day…we was talking…I don't know whether it
is the situation you sort of meet…you explain things to them and you
sort of…well this day he came in and we was talking about different
things. We was talking about colour TVs. Can you remember…? And
he turned round and you know he says until not long ago he thought
that in the 1930s and 1940s everything was black and white, because
that is how it was portrayed on television, and it was only a few months
ago that he had actually learnt that it wasn't, it was just the fact there
was only black and white televisions, you know!
Mother of Harry, 20 years, BSL

The stories are recounted because they are unusual and striking. They are
not simply an account of particular misunderstandings, but illustrate how
information may not be available to deaf people. As a consequence of this,
deaf people may sometimes be seen as ignorant, as lacking understanding

Table 9.1. *Language skills and preferred language*

	BSL	SSE	Oral
General comprehension			
Average score	6.5	6.3	7.2
Range	1–8	4–8	2–8
Complex comprehension			
Average score	3.8	5.9	5.3
Range	1–8	4–8	1–8
Complex answers			
Average score	5.1	7.5	5.4
Range	1–8	4–8	2–8

or even egocentric. There is a lack of awareness of the importance of the dissemination of information at formal and informal levels. The implications of this are considered later in the chapter.

Preferred language

Throughout this book we have described the young people in terms of their preferred language rather than their hearing loss, which would have been the more conventional decision. Preferred language was seen as the more appropriate distinction, as representing the young person's identity in a way they related more to their own choice. As was shown in Chapter 1, preferred language has a relationship with hearing loss, though not a complete one. Not surprisingly, preferred language related to a number of social aspects of the young people's lives. Those who went to Deaf Club, identified with the Deaf community and had mainly deaf friends were more likely to be BSL users. Those who had mostly hearing friends and socialised within the hearing world were more likely to be oral. Other factors did not show a relationship – the degree of independence, personality factors, obtaining and staying in work, and extent of their social life.

Overall, the level of language of those who were oral was better than those using BSL in terms of the various comprehension and expression scales described in Chapter 1, as is shown in Table 9.1. This is not of course to endorse the idea that the oral approach is better. The two languages did not have equal status in the lives of the young people, who were offered only oral methods in their early lives. In addition, the only grammar school for deaf children in the country takes only those pupils who will benefit from an oral education, so this higher level of education is available only to those who have oral skills. It should be noted that in all categories some BSL users scored in the highest category, affirming that BSL is in no way a barrier to good communication skills. What factors contribute to whether or not a young person will prefer BSL or English as their first language is difficult to establish, particularly given the bias to oral language when the children were young. While we cannot show what would have happened if all the young people had been offered English and BSL from the start, we ourselves are confident that many more would have achieved full linguistic competence with positive ensuing consequences.

We do know that the young people who grew up to use BSL or SSE were more likely to have families who used gesture and who approved of the use of gesture when they were young. The type of school and attitude to signing at school showed a relationship with preferred language. For most of those attending mainstream schools at secondary stage, the preferred language was oral (ten oral, one BSL). The situation for those attending schools for the deaf is less clear, because some were (and still are) strictly oral. Of those attending schools for the deaf at secondary stage, 22 became BSL users, ten SSE users and nine were oral. Based on parental reports of school approach, more than one-third of BSL users (12/31) and half (6/13) of SSE users attended schools at the secondary stage with positive attitudes to sign language. No-one who went to such a school had spoken English as their preferred language later on. Most of those whose preferred language was oral attended schools that were oral in approach (26/30), although these were also attended by a small proportion of BSL and SSE users (2/31 BSL users and 5/13 SSE users). (Young people not represented in this analysis attended schools that accepted signing but did not encourage it, or where the approach changed during their secondary school career.) It would be difficult, however, to cite a causal relationship here. The extent to which the parental or child language preference influenced the choice of school, or the attitude of the school influenced later language preference, is difficult to determine.

Gender differences

We have isolated gender as an issue for consideration, as a number of differences emerged, despite the fact that we did not set out specifically to explore them. There was a tendency for young men to be among the lowest achievers. All of those with limited language skills, and all of those who could not read, write or do numerical tasks were male. As one might assume, there was considerable overlap between these groups.

A further difference occurred in preferred language, for while the split between English (oral or SSE) and BSL was similar for young men and young women, there was a difference within the English group. Many more women than men preferred SSE (11 women and only two men) and we have suggested that this indicates a higher priority for communication by many young women compared with men.

No clear differences emerged in factors of personality or degree of independence. However, we were interested in this study to uncover gender differences in the area of social life and friends. In brief, in both choice of partners and friends, young women were more likely to prefer deaf people, seemingly indicating a higher priority being given to communication. In contrast, some young men appeared more instrumental in their wishes and wanted hearing company. In terms of friendship, this may reflect different social activities of men and women, the women preferring to engage in conversation, while the men seemed more likely to take part in group activities where the communication demands were more predictable and less complex. In partnerships, however, the wish for young men was more pragmatic, and some explicitly suggested that a hearing partner was more desirable as she could interface with the hearing world.

Attitudes to deaf people

In the first study, the attitudes of others to the deaf child and the family were a significant issue. About three-quarters of parents then felt there was a general lack of understanding of deafness. With older sons and daughters it was not such an issue, the deafness had become part of the family's experience. The novelty had gone and parents had become more accustomed to talking about their situation.

In addition, it was felt that attitudes to deafness had changed, in particular, because it had become more visible on television through specialist programmes, but also through signed interpretation of some mainstream programmes. The vast majority of parents (65, 79%) felt that attitudes had changed in the period between the two interviews, although only 14 (17%) perceived any major development and most (46, 56%) saw the changes as limited.

By and large the attitude of hearing people to deaf people is apathy and lack of understanding. The medical profession was often singled out as lacking awareness, GPs often requiring parents to attend with their deaf sons and daughters, and hospital staff not realising the difficulties for deaf patients in the hospital situation. In contrast, driving instructors were a notable exception and seemed to regard teaching deaf people to drive as a challenge.

An area that was seen as particularly destructive in terms of negative attitudes or ignorance was that of employment, where attitudes of employers, but also those of the professionals employed to assist young people in obtaining work and training, were seen as particularly inadequate, resulting in limited work opportunities, inadequate training and lack of promotion opportunities, leading to underemployment. There were some notable exceptions where young deaf people had received excellent support advice and opportunities, but these only served to illustrate what could be done, rather than excuse the overall picture.

Developing independence

A particular issue, significant because of the age of the young people interviewed, was their developing independence. The late teens and early twenties are the period when most people establish independence from their families, both financially and also in terms of setting up their own homes. This was the wish of the majority of young deaf people and the parents interviewed for this book. In many respects many had achieved this. However, the issues already discussed – language and communication and access to information – could have an inhibiting effect here. Parents were often involved in the young people's lives in ways that both felt were not ideal. They could be asked to facilitate communication or assist in arrangements with friends and colleagues of the young person. They could take a major role in obtaining employment. They often went to great lengths to explain financial and other matters when the information was not readily available in an accessible form elsewhere. Many of these concerns would be resolved by changes in attitudes to deafness and the better provision of technical equipment, as is discussed later in this chapter. It is to the credit of many of the young people and their families that they had achieved the independence they had, in their living, working and social lives.

VARYING PERSPECTIVES

Parents' and young people's views

For the most part, there was considerable agreement between the young people's and parents' perspectives on their experiences. Both parents and young people presented a complex picture and inevitably there were differences, although overall the main feature was agreement. However, there were a few areas where differences emerged, which are of intrinsic interest, because of how they illustrate differing perspectives.

The first area of difference was in education. While the majority of young people were happiest at secondary school, most dissatisfaction was felt by parents at this stage. We felt this to be clearly a consequence of different perceptions. Deaf children may appear to do well at primary school, where it may be easy to copy what others do, to appear to understand. However, often their language and communication had not developed and they themselves were confused and worried. By the secondary stage, the young people seemed to have more understanding of what was happening and a greater sense of their own identity. Friendships with peers were important and for many of them their relationships with their deaf friends made them more confident. However, at this stage the parents became much more aware of the implications of deafness and the difference between their sons and daughters and other young people of the same age. In addition, they were starting to think, with concern, about the future.

A second area was that of friendships and relationships. Parents seemed to take a more pessimistic view of their sons' and daughters' social lives than did the young people themselves. Here we were aware that the relationships were being viewed in a different context. For the most part, the parental concept of social life was a hearing view, involving regular contact with a number of people, most of whom were likely to live locally. Many hearing young people at this age develop friendships at work. Many of the deaf young people saw their friends less regularly but travelled all over the country to meet up with people, and belonged to a vast network of relationships. Many compared their own experience favourably with their perception of the relationships of hearing young people, which they saw as being more limited. They were, however, less likely to make friends at work.

A third, though less tangible, difference was in the attitude of the young deaf person to their deafness. For most of them, by the time of the interview, deafness was an intrinsic part of themselves. For the parents, even for those who felt they had accepted the deafness, almost all still thought in terms of the hearing person that might have been, a notion that was alien to the deaf young people. It may be, though evidence here is circumstantial, that the fact that parents were less likely to see their sons and daughters as associated with Deaf Clubs than were the deaf young people themselves, is relevant here.

Early experience and later development

Comparing early parental accounts with the later interviews provided an opportunity to review those aspects of early behaviour that were linked to later consequences and those that were not, and some aspects of the child's behaviour or preferences were indicators of later behaviour. In terms of preferred language, children who were to grow up to use sign language showed an early preference for gesture in communication and their spoken language was less well developed. It was the actual use of gesture more than the parents' approval or disapproval of gesture that was important in this respect. Those who preferred SSE later in life were more similar in their early behaviours to those who used BSL, rather than to those who were later oral.

Later hearing-aid use also showed a relationship with early behaviour. Interestingly, the strongest relationship was not with how much the aid was worn early on but whether or not the child tolerated or resisted the aid. Therefore, the child's early preferences, rather than imposed use of hearing aids, were the clearest indicator of later behaviour.

In both these areas, a note of caution should be sounded. Even when there is a significant relationship, there are always exceptions. There were those who had a preference for oral language later on, yet preferred gesture early and whose language was slow in developing or alternatively, those who were BSL users later on whose early communication was through spoken language. Although the relationship exists for the population as a whole, the individual child can be different.

Some personal and social aspects of the young people also showed a relationship with behaviours in their earlier life. Those who were described by their parents as unhappy or varying between happy and unhappy as young adults were more likely to have had many temper tantrums as a young child. Many tantrums as a child was also a feature of those young people who were seen by their parents as easily bored as young adults. In addition, the majority of young people who made friends easily had good social skills as a child, according to the parents' responses to a number of questions then. However, there was not a predictive relationship based on the amount of contact they had with other children when the young people were children.

Consistency over time

A consequence of re-interviewing parents after some considerable time was that it provided an opportunity to consider the way in which interview accounts are constructed and the reliability and validity of interview accounts. This has not been developed in detail in the book, but there are clearly a number of reasons why such material should be of interest, some extending beyond the concerns of the present study. Firstly, it is important to understand how parents actually represent the past and the context of both stable and varying accounts. Secondly, having a deaf child puts parents in a situation that is both unfamiliar and often disturbing in some way, and it is useful to understand the process by which parents make sense of this for themselves. Thirdly, there is a practical concern with more general implications. Many disabling conditions become apparent only as the child grows older, yet it is often important to know about aspects of the child's early history. In trying to describe the aetiology and early course of particular conditions, such as autism, it is important to know those factors that may influence the reports parents make about the child's early behaviour and development.

We have seen in Chapter 8, the moment of diagnosis was remembered particularly vividly, often to the actual words used. Interestingly, although diagnosis was almost always remembered with clarity, in a number of areas and for a number of reasons, there were changes over the period of the interviews. For example, there was remarkable consistency in the cause of deafness when specific causes were given at both interviews, but there was a change over those that were initially reported to be of unknown aetiology. Where mothers specified a particular cause at both interviews, the only change was for one child whose deafness was initially reported to be due to prematurity, but later said to be due to the rhesus factor. This could well have been due to extra information received later. For half (40/80, 50%) for whom the question could be put, the cause was unknown at the earlier age, but this was only the case for 27 (34%) at the later age. For most of these the cause was given as genetic, but other common causes of childhood deafness – rubella, meningitis, prematurity and the rhesus factor – were also mentioned. It may be that new information emerged after the first interview. However, it is clear in talking to parents, that being able to identify a cause for a disability is very important. It may well be that in the time between the interviews, they discussed, asked questions, collected information and evolved some explanation which made sense of their child's disability to them.

Two main areas of concern in the first study were difficulties with sleeping and temper tantrums. In both these areas, deaf children showed differences from hearing children of the same age. Parents were asked in the later interview if these had been issues in childhood. In both these areas, there were changes in reports of behaviour over time. Of the 34 who were reported to wake often by parents in the earlier interview, only 20 (59%) were later reported to have had sleep problems. The largest group (44) reported tantrums at both ages, but of the 18 that were reported in the later interview as not having had tantrums as a child, nearly half (eight) were reported early on as having tantrums.

Clearly, one aspect of this is that parents were describing a longer time scale. It may be that, in the case of the move from no problem to problems, there was a change in behaviour since the earlier interview. However, it could also be that the happenings were seen in a much wider context and re-interpreted or reconstructed in terms of a much broader perspective. Bedtime problems and temper tantrums, which seemed overwhelming at the time, could later on be a small and irrelevant part of the child's development and of no lasting significance.

There is another factor that appears to play a part. Later experiences could ameliorate or modify the understanding of earlier ones. An example of this can be seen in the following two accounts of children starting school.

(Did it take him long to settle?)

No it didn't – he settled very well. We had him home for the first weekend like, and took him back. Well, he seemed a bit upset then like, but after that he seemed keen to get back.
Mother of Ivan, 4 years (part of research for DCF, quote not included there)

It was terrible for the first two years – until he got to about five. He'd go screaming. Then they used to get them standing up in the window so you could wave to them – well, it used to be heart-breaking – seeing them there with bottom lips going.
Mother of Ivan, 21 years, BSL

They're very pleased for you to inquire, but I don't think they like you to see life there. I don't know, I might be wrong, but that's the impression I get. I stayed the first days, I put him to bed at night, I stayed in the hotel opposite, put him to bed myself at night. But the headmaster wouldn't let me stay the next day, and I badly wanted to, just to see the routine and what they did, but he said, 'No, ten o'clock's long enough'. So I went and said goodbye to him at ten o'clock. It was terrible.
Mother of Robert, 5 years (DCF, p. 141)

Interviewer: Did you like…School?
Oh yes, I did, very much. Got on very well with the staff and everybody.
Interviewer: Was there anything about it that you particularly liked?

I liked the atmosphere. The friendliness, particularly the nursery where the children have to be made to feel secure. That's the most important thing, I think, at that age. Security.
Interviewer: Anything you disliked?
I can't think of anything at the moment. No.
Mother of Robert, 22 years, BSL

Ivan was never really happy at school and left at the earliest opportunity, whereas Robert went on to be very successful, stayed at the same school throughout, and became head boy.

Thus our interview studies have revealed a number of areas in which early and later accounts vary. Sometimes this reflects the evolving accounts of parents, sometimes a change in attitudes over time, and sometimes the context in which the account is developed had changed. We would not suggest that these parents are deliberately being dishonest, or that their memories are faulty when the accounts differ. Rather, the frame in which they are interpreting them changes and gives a different emphasis to the story. The issue is not the 'truth' of memories, and it is not clear that we should favour early accounts over later ones. What is important is to understand the way in which parents construct, under varying circumstances, their accounts of their children's childhood. (See Gregory 1991*b* for a fuller discussion of this topic.) This issue is also discussed in Appendix III, which considers the interview as a research tool.

IMPLICATIONS

The role of sign language

One of the main issues confronting the young deaf person and the family is language and communication. Most of the young people had been brought up, at least in the early stages of their lives, using an oral approach. Most parents and young people felt they should have been told about sign language, that it should have been at least offered to them as a possibility. Where parents learnt to sign, the young people viewed this positively, and therefore the suggestion that deaf children should be introduced to sign language early on to facilitate language and communication seems attractive. We ourselves feel that this is the obvious and proper conclusion from our interviews with parents and young people. This is not to say that all those born deaf, or becoming deaf early in life should have British Sign Language as their first or main language, but that the introduction to signing early in life will facilitate development in a number of areas. We are not ourselves convinced by the arguments that suggest that the introduction of sign language can inhibit spoken language, but rather are of the opinion that it can facilitate it. The enormous benefits of good language skills for personal development should not be ignored.

However, to introduce sign language is not without problems. It would require parents to become competent in a second language at the time their child was diagnosed, and learning the baby register of a language (the simplified form used by adults with babies and young children) can be more complex than simply acquiring the language. All the problems that are already found in the oral system where the mother is the only or main communicator may be exacerbated and the pair could be isolated within the family. It would create an environment where the child could communicate, but may not extend the range of people with whom they could communicate. Only in the most exceptional families does it seem that the extended family, grandparents and so on, would learn to sign. A number of projects have been developed where deaf people go into families and teach sign language. While this is usually received with enthusiasm by the families, the long-term results have yet to be established.

It should be said at the outset that no-one wanted sign language to the exclusion of English, and a significant proportion of deaf young people and their parents felt that speech intelligibility was important. Most of the young people did use signs and speech. Most parents and young people saw both languages as important. Many felt that they had been failed in a number of respects, in not being introduced to signing at an earlier stage. They felt that more work on speech was required, even if only to say a few words well.

Their priorities probably differed from those of the professionals involved with whom they had contact. From the interviews, it seemed that in the early years communication was seen as of the utmost importance, however it was achieved, whereas later on the ability to communicate with hearing people as well as deaf people seemed a priority. This is a more pragmatic view than that of many professionals. They tend to stress oral speech throughout the child's life even at the early stages when it can limit communication. Alternatively, they favour sign language and literacy, but feel that the ability to speak is of secondary or minor importance. Many parents were very disappointed with the quality of their son's or daughter's speech. For many parents, intelligible speech had a high priority and often they wanted speech to be developed, not necessarily as the main language for communication, but trained in specific areas to facilitate interaction in the hearing world. One father suggested that the ability to articulate one hundred words clearly could make all the difference.

The research has shown that most families see sign language as important and feel that they should be given the best information possible about it. Ways need to be evolved to introduce this as early and effectively as possible for those families who wish to sign. However, this should not be at the expense of spoken language skills and strategies to communicate in the hearing world. It may well be, though, that early linguistic competence may provide the basis for later ease of communication.

Education

On the topic of education we were constantly impressed with the measured arguments the parents and young people proffered, which often contrasted with the more entrenched positions held by a large number of professionals. Parents could see reason for integration and for segregation, for using signing and for focusing on oral skills, yet their overall position was more pragmatic. They wanted their sons and daughters to be prepared for the hearing world and to take their place in it, but did not necessarily see integration as providing the best means of achieving this. Most felt that speech intelligibility was an important asset, but also felt that to deny sign language as a means of providing a high standard of education was wrong. Many of them felt that they and their sons and daughters had been failed by the provision that had been available to them.

The conclusion that we ourselves draw from this is that most of the young people would have benefited from a system of education that valued both English and BSL, a bilingual approach. Without sign language, many of the young people had been deprived of full access to the curriculum, as well as the variety of social experiences that would have been facilitated by such linguistic competence. However, an approach that only valued signing would have limited the young person's opportunities within the majority hearing world, for work, training, social contacts and leisure. Literacy, an essential component of life in modern societies, is dependent upon English. In addition, and perhaps contrary to the views of some members of the Deaf community, where appropriate, good intelligible speech is a legitimate goal for education. We ourselves see this to be compatible with a bilingual approach to education.

The young people, too, presented us with a new perspective on education. Although a significant number of them favoured special education, a large number also wanted integration, to be educated within a hearing world, although not in the way currently practised. This was clearly an area to which the young people had given a great deal of thought, because here they were at their most innovative, and they stressed the need for integration in large numbers, half the school being deaf and half hearing, if possible.

The other view that surprised us was a complete turn on its head of traditional orthodoxy. Usually, it is felt that integration is suitable for young deaf children as the language demands are seen as less complex, but as children get to secondary stage and the linguistic demands are greater, special school may be required. Only a few young people raised this issue, but those who did stressed the need for a peer group for the young deaf child to facilitate communication and develop their own sense of identity. From their own experience they explained that much unhappiness could be felt at an early age, but may not be easily expressed and the young child might not have the resources to cope with it. However, at secondary stage the emphasis changes, and integration seems more desirable. The young person needs to learn to cope with the hearing world, needs to have contact with a wide range of people of his or her own peer group and could have developed the language and confidence to cope. It was also felt by some that a higher standard of education could be maintained in the hearing schools.

School–work transition

As in most other studies of deaf young people and adults, this study revealed significant difficulties in the area of training and employment. Moore & Beazley (1991) found in their study of deaf young people that few had received proper vocational advice. Kyle & Allsop (1982) reported significant underemployment of deaf adults in the UK and Jones & Pullen (1990) suggested that this is the case throughout the European Community.

We have already suggested that part of this may be due to attitudes of employers and professionals. However, we would further suggest that many deaf people are not fully aware of work and training and without this information are unable to develop and realise their aspirations. We have argued elsewhere (Sheldon, Gregory & Bishop, 1990) that 'in order for deaf young people to take responsibility for their career choices, they need to be exposed to an environment which encourages the development of ideas and opinions: and to learn from the experience of others'.

We feel that if deaf young people are to have equal opportunities at work, they must have equal access to further education and training.

Currently they are under-represented in further and higher education. A report by the Royal National Institute of the Deaf (RNID; Daniels & Corlett, 1990) suggests that rather than the 0.2% of the population in higher education being deaf as would be expected, it is probably less than 0.1%, though the absence of available figures make the comparison difficult to ascertain. This report goes on to make a number of useful recommendations, including admissions monitoring and adequate funding for support, which would be endorsed by the findings from this research. Support that was provided at colleges for the young people was erratic and inadequate. In the 1980s there was little consistent provision for deaf students in further education and little specialist training available for professionals in this area. As Green & Nickerson (1992) point out: 'It was becoming clear to LSDs (lecturers with students who are deaf) and TODs (Teachers of the Deaf) by 1985 that they were faced with a daunting situation wherein the scope of work and expectations of them far outstripped the training and professional guidance and support available to them at a personal level'. It is to be hoped that support grants to deaf students, introduced in 1990, will go some way to ameliorate the situation. However, the capacity of deaf students to benefit from education and training will still depend on their linguistic competence and, as we have seen from the group considered in this book, this remains an issue to be addressed.

Access to information

We have argued in this book that access to information is as critical an issue for deaf people as is language and communication. Technological support is important here, both in terms of aids devised specifically for deaf people and technological advances within the wider community. Two-thirds of the young people interviewed benefited from their hearing aids, and other equipment was useful to varying degrees. Text telephones are a significant development and are becoming more so as institutions and companies see them as necessary equipment. Subtitles on television were mentioned as a major development. Because of their importance, not just for entertainment purposes but in facilitating access to information, it seems clear to us that they should be seen as part of the general provision of the television companies. Access to information is as significant as access to buildings and any equal opportunities policy needs to address this. It is to be hoped that the launch of the Royal National Institute for the Deaf check 'Louder than words' campaign in January 1993, after the research interviews had been completed, will go some way to ameliorate the situation. The campaign seeks a commitment on the part of large organisations to make their services more readily accessible to deaf people and the RNID have developed a 'Deaf Awareness Pack' to support this initiative.

BSL users require interpreters in order to interface with the hearing world. Many deaf people who communicate orally in face-to-face situations still require, or benefit from, interpreters in larger groups and their participation may be dependent on such provision. Since the interviews were completed, The Commission of Enquiry into Human Aids to Communication (1992), set up by four of the major Deaf organisations, has made its report, 'Communication is Your Responsibility'. This report makes many recommendations to improve communication support for deaf people, which are being put to Government and private organisations.

We have been interested to note that developments to make services and information more available to hearing people have also been of benefit to deaf people. Self-service shopping is an instance in point. It also seems significant that travelling by air could be easier for the deaf young people than travelling by bus or train. Airports need to meet the needs of people using a variety of languages, and thus have developed clear ways of presenting information through a variety of modalities.

However, as well as technical equipment, the attitudes of the general public to deaf people is a critical factor. Society needs to recognise that 'deaf' does not mean 'daft', and that deaf people, regardless of whether they choose to use spoken or sign language, are potentially competent members of society. If their equal rights are recognised, they will be able to participate more fully in society.

The Deaf community

Some readers of this book may be disappointed that there is not more discussion of Deaf identity, Deaf pride and the Deaf community. However, this reflects the findings of the interviews. The Deaf community in the UK sees itself as a strong identifiable group and many members would describe themselves as belonging to a linguistic and cultural minority group. It is thus surprising how little this community had impinged on the lives of the young deaf people. While the majority had attended Deaf Clubs at some time or the other, and for many it was an important part of their social lives, few seemed to see themselves as part of a community of Deaf people. While a significant number of the deaf young people had a Deaf identity, in that they saw their deafness as an integral part of their personality, they rarely mentioned being part of a community of Deaf people in this context. Discussions of Deaf issues was rare in the interviews, although it did emerge in the group discussions. It was the impression of the interviewer that the majority had only minimal knowledge of Deaf issues and some had no understanding at all. At the time of the interviews only seven (11%) belonged to any of the major national Deaf organisations.

The Deaf community would seem to have a role for both parents and young people. The need for the Deaf community to be involved with deaf children and young people has been discussed by The British Deaf Association in recent years. At their Rothesay Congress (1986), they passed a motion that stated:

> This Congress recognises that future developments of the deaf community requires the full participation of deaf children and young people. Congress therefore urges BDA branches, regions and the Executive Council to consider initiatives which will create opportunities for the fuller involvement of deaf children and young people in the life of the community   (Cited in Grant, 1990)

We feel that the findings from this research imply a significant and increasing role for the Deaf community in the area of sign language and in attitudes to hearing families with deaf members, and for deaf young people.

The advice from parents

The consequences of the deafness of the young person for the parents are too numerous to reiterate at this point. They could feel their health, social life and work had been affected by the deafness, although they were more likely to report this when their sons and daughters were young than when they were young adults. While some parents described consequences for their marriage, the actual statistics on marriage breakdown and divorce did not seem to vary greatly from those that would be expected of the population in general. Most parents mentioned some pressures and strains, though many also commented on an increased sensitivity and general insights that they had developed.

We did ask the parents what advice they would give to other parents in the same position.

I would fight hard for all the things that – to make people aware of your child. If they are sight impaired, then they have to have glasses. Deafness is something you can't observe and therefore you have to

make people more aware that your child needs extra help and attention.
When your child is deaf or whatever, you will do far more for your child
than you would yourself. I think it's just making people more aware.
Mother of Louise, 22 years, oral

I don't think I was ever told anything, but I do think – not to think it's
the end of the world, you know, and to go to a Deaf Club somewhere
and just see the fact they can actually grow up into adults, who have a
contribution to make, you know. () I happened to be there one Friday
night when all the youth club people came and there was a disco in the
basement, and we went down; I just wanted to see teenage deaf people,
you know, and it was sitting there, looking at them and I thought, they
do grow up. They do grow into people who laugh and you know, there
is a life.
Mother of Veronica, 21 years, SSE

Any means of communication is viable. You have to forget the
embarrassment. The child must have someone that understands. It
doesn't matter what the world thinks. Get in touch with anybody who
has had any experience with deaf people as near to your child's age as
you can. You need to know that ordinary deaf children survive. They
can do anything they set their minds to. It's not disabling. If they really
want to they can do it.
Mother of Nicky, 21 years, SSE

This mother describes how she has spoken about being deaf to her son.

If you go through life with a chip on your shoulder expecting things to
happen because you are deaf, you can't have that attitude. You've got to
fit into life as it is. You've got to make a choice if you're a deaf person:
are you going to be an oral deaf, a signing deaf, or what? Do you flit in
and out? Ray has chosen to be in the middle. He flits in and out of the
others. He is happiest in his oral, he goes into deaf signing and he goes
into the hearing and that is when he's happiest. Are they going to have
nothing to do with Deaf culture, and go and be as integrated into the
hearing world as possible, or are they going to be where Ray is, where he
feels most comfortable?
Mother of Ray, 21 years, oral

Table 9.2. *Future hopes of the deaf young people*

	Young men		Young women		Total	
	Number	%	Number	%	Number	%
Family-related	3	9	10	37	13	22
Work-related	7	22	4	14	11	19
Material goods	5	16	4	14	9	15
Success/happiness	7	21	0	0	7	12
Travel	3	9	3	11	6	10
Other	7	22	5	19	12	20
Don't know	0	0	1	4	1	2

THE FUTURE

***I am waiting for all my dreams to come true, but I don't know what
my dreams are yet***

The final question in the interviews with the deaf young people was, 'What
do you hope for in the future?' We hoped this would enable us to end the
interview on a positive note. In our analysis we have taken the first or
dominant response, although in about one-third of all answers they
elaborated on more than one theme. The majority of those able to answer
(46/59, 78%) fell into the categories of wishes concerning family, work,
material success, happiness or travel, although there were gender differences, as is shown in Table 9.2. The young men gave priority to work or a
more general notion of success, whereas the women were more likely to
talk of their wishes for a family. Those in the 'other' category ranged from
world peace, to travel into space, to wanting to pass the driving test, a very
immediate concern for the young man involved. And as our heading quote
describes, one just wanted his dreams to come true, although he was not
yet sure what his dreams were.

Most of the parents (73, 89%) had worries about the future, relationships (26, 32%) work (16, 20%) and both work and relationships (24,
29%), though some were unconcerned.

> *No, not really, he knows right from wrong, the birds and the bees, and
> he has passed his driving test and he has a job. We are very optimistic.
> Mother of Harry, 20 years, BSL*

Having begun the book with the account of Isabel and her family, perhaps
we should end with this quote from her mother as she looks to the future.

But it is like I said earlier. I could never see the day when Isabel would be the person she is today () but maybe if you come to me again, if I am still here God willing, in another 20 years, maybe I will be saying the same thing to you again. I could never see the day when Isabel would be a mother and bringing up children. This is what it is like when you have got a deaf child. I suppose it is what it is like when you have got any child that is handicapped. You can never see that much ahead. So if you come back in 20 years' time I will be saying, 'I could never see the day when Isabel would be a mother and bringing up these kids'. You know, you can't see that much ahead.

Mother of Isabel

REFERENCES

Brennan, M. (1976). Can deaf children acquire language? *British Deaf News*, February, Supplement.

Central Statistical Office (1992). *Social Trends*, **22**. London HMSO.

Commission of Enquiry into Human Aids to Communication (1992). *Communication is Your Responsibility*. London: Panel of Four.

Conrad, R. (1979). *The Deaf School Child*. London: Harper Row.

Courtenay, G. (1989). *The Youth Cohort Study of England and Wales. Notes on Young People aged 16–19*. Prepared for The Prince's Trust, Social and Community Planning Research.

Dale, D. (1967). *Deaf Children at Home and School*. London: University of London Press.

Daniels, S. & Corlett, S. (1990). *Deaf Students in Higher Education: A Survey of Policy and Practice*. Research Report 9. London: Royal National Institute for the Deaf.

Denmark, J., Rodda, M., Abel, R., Skelton, U., Eldridge, R.W., Warren, F. & Gordon, A. (1979). *A Word in Deaf Ears*. London: Royal National Institute for the Deaf.

Denton, D.M. (1976). *Remarks in Support of a System of Total Communication for Deaf Children*, Communication Symposium. Frederick: Maryland School for the Deaf.

Department of Education and Science, DES (1981), Circular 8/81, Education Act 1981. London: HMSO.

Department of Health and Social Security (DHSS) (1988) *'Say it Again': Contemporary Social Work Practice with People who are Deaf and Hard of Hearing*. London: Social Services Inspectorate, Department of Health and Social Security.

Dunn, J. & Kendrick, C. (1982). *Siblings*. London: Grant McIntyre.

Finkelstein, V. (1991). 'We' are not disabled 'You' are. In *Constructing Deafness*, ed. S. Gregory & G. Hartley. London: Pinter Publishers.

Grant, B. (1990). *The Deaf Advance: A History of the British Deaf Association*. Edinburgh: The Pentland Press.

Green, C. & Nickerson, W. (1992). *The Rise of the Communicator: A Perspective on Post 16 Education and Training for Deaf People*. Moonshine Publishers.

Gregory, S. (1976). *The Deaf Child and His Family*. London: George Allen and Unwin. Re-issued as *Deaf Children and Their Families* (1995). Cambridge: Cambridge University Press.

  (1991*a*). Challenging motherhood: mothers and their deaf children, in *Motherhood; Meanings, Practices and Ideologies*, ed. A. Phoenix, A., Woolett & E. Lloyd. London: Sage.

  (1991*b*). *Remembering Past Events: The Parent's Tale*. Paper presented to the British Psychological Society Developmental Section Conference, Cambridge, September 1991.

  (1993). The language and culture of deaf people: implications for education, in *Language, Culture and Education*, ed. M.C. Beveridge & G. Reddiford. Clevedon: Multilingual Matters, also in *Language and Education*, vol. 6, pp. 2–4 (1992).

Gregory, S. & Bishop, J. (1991). The mainstreaming of primary age deaf children in *Constructing Deafness*, ed. S. Gregory & G. Hartley. London: Pinter Press.

Harris, A. (1971). *Handicapped and Impaired in Great Britain*. London: Her Majesty's Stationery Office.

Hartley, G. (1988). Aspects of the Home Care of Deaf Children of Deaf Parents. Unpublished PhD thesis, University of Nottingham, Nottingham.

Jackson, P. (1986). *The Allan Hayhurst Research Fellowship Report*, presented to the British Deaf Association Congress, Rothesay, Isle of Bute.

  (1991). *Britain's Deaf Heritage*. Edinburgh: Pentland Press.

Jones, L. & Pullen, G. (1990). *Inside We Are All Equal: A Social Policy Survey of Deaf People in the European Community*. London: European Community Regional Secretariat of the World Federation of the Deaf.

Kyle, J. & Allsop, L. (1982). *Deaf People and the Community. Final Report to the Nuffield Foundation*. Bristol: School of Education.

Ling, A.H. (1968). Advice for parents of young deaf children: how to begin. *Volta Review*, **12**, (70).

Lynas, W. (1986). *Integrating the Handicapped into Ordinary Schools: A Study of Hearing Impaired Pupils*. London: Croom Helm.

Lysons, K. (1979). *The Development of Local Voluntary Societies for Adult Deaf Persons in England*. British Deaf News, Carlisle.

Meherali, R. (1984). The Deaf Asian Child and His Family. Unpublished thesis submitted in part requirement for MA, Child Developmental Research Unit, University of Nottingham, Nottingham.

Moore, M. & Beazley, S. (1991). The Post School Reflections of Young Deaf People. Unpublished report, Manchester, Manchester Polytechnic, Department of Psychology and Speech Pathology.

National Deaf Children's Society (1971). *Annual Report and Accounts (1970–1971)*. London: National Deaf Children's Society.

(1982). *Year Book and Annual Report (1981–82)*. London: National Deaf Children's Society.

(1987). *For all Deaf Children (Annual Report and Accounts 1986/87)*. London: National Deaf Children's Society.

Newson, J. & Newson, E. (1963). *Infant Care in the Urban Community*. London: George Allen and Unwin.

(1968). *Four Years Old in an Urban Community*, London: Allen and Unwin.

Noller, P. & Callan, V. (1991). *The Adolescent in the Family*. London: Routledge Kegan Paul.

Oliver, M. (1989). Conductive education: if it wasn't so sad it would be funny. *Disability Handicap and Society*, 4, (2).

(1990). *The Politics of Disablement*. London: MacMillan.

Padden, C. & Humphries, T. (1988). *Deaf in America: Voices from a Culture*. London: Harvard University Press.

Phoenix, S. (1988). *An Interim Report on a Pilot Survey of Deaf Adults in Northern Ireland with Detailed Reference to their Educational Experience, Employment and Social Situation*. London: Royal National Institute for the Deaf.

Rodda, M. (1970). *The Hearing Impaired School Leaver*. London: University of London Press.

Rodda M. & Grove, C. (1987). *Language, Cognition and Deafness*. London: Lawrence Erlbaum Associates.

Sainsbury, S. (1986). *Deaf Worlds*. London: Hutchinson.

Sharma, A. & Love, D. (1991). *A Change in Approach: A Report on the Experience of Deaf People from Black and Ethnic Minority Communities*. London: Royal Association in Aid of Deaf People.

Sheldon, L., Gregory, S. & Bishop, J. (1990). The transition from school to work. Paper presented at the *17th International Congress on the Education of the Deaf*, Rochester, USA, July.

Silo, J. (work in progress). *The Role of Deaf Teachers in the Education of Deaf Children*. MPhil thesis (in preparation), The Open University.

Voysey, M. (1975). *A Constant Burden: the Reconstitution of Family Life*. London: Routledge Kegan Paul.

Wood, D., Wood, H. & Howarth, P. (1983). Mathematical abilities of deaf school leavers. *British Journal of Developmental Psychology*, 1.

Guided interview schedule

PARENTS' SCHEDULE

Date of Interview   Interviewer

N's name and address

               Tel

Date of Birth   Age

Mother's Name and Address (if different)

               Tel

FACT SHEET

(a) Previous family details

(b) Present family context

	Father	Mother	Sibling	Sibling	Sibling	Sibling	Anyone living with family
Name							
Natural/step							

	Father	Mother	Sibling	Sibling	Sibling	Sibling	Anyone living with family
Sex							
Age							
Disability							
At home							
School/ college/work							
Present at interview							
Children							

(c) Other information

Part 1

DIAGNOSIS

1. I wonder if first of all I can get an idea of how deaf N is? Can he/she hear anything at all?

2. Can he/she hear if you shout/talk normally close to him/her when he/she's not wearing his/her hearing aid?

    Probe   *And what about with his/her aid?*

3. Has he/she been deaf since birth as far as you know?

4. Do you know the cause of N's deafness?

5. Can you tell me when you were first told that N might be deaf? (Who told you?)

6. Have you been told how deaf he/she is?

7. Had you any idea before that there was something wrong?

    Probe   If yes – *What made you think that?*

    Did you tell anyone else what you thought?

8. When ... told you about N, what did he/she actually say to you?

    Probe   *How did you feel about it?*

9. Did you take it in then? – and your husband/wife (did he/she take it in?)

10. How do you feel about the way you were told?

11. *If appropriate* – What is the best time to be told this sort of thing?

    Probe   *Is it better to be told as soon as possible or after some time?*

12. When was the last time N's hearing was assessed?

    Probe   *By whom?*

    Details?

13. What sort of hearing aid does N have nowadays?

    Probe   *Does he/she wear it? Are there times when he/she chooses not to wear it?*

    Is he/she pleased with it?

14. Does N have any other pieces of equipment which he/she uses?

    Probe   *Ceefax/subtitles/teletext?*

    Flashing doorbell?

    Telephone aids?

    Baby alarms?

    Hearing dog?

    Vibrating pillow?

    Computer? (and how does he/she use it?)

    Other?

SCHOOL EXPERIENCE

15. I'd like to trace N's school experiences from pre-school right up to the point where he/she left secondary school. Could you tell me a little about N's school experiences?

16. When did he/she start full-time school?

17. Did he/she go to a nursery or anything like that?

18. Did ... school have any strong ideas about the way N should communicate?

    Probe *What did you feel about that?*

19. Did N like...school?

20. And what about you?

    Probe *Was there anything you particularly liked?*

    Was there anything you particularly disliked?

21. After...school where did he/she go?

22. Did you choose that school or was it suggested?

23. And did they have particular views on communication?

24. Did N like...school?

25. And what about you?

    Probe *Was there anything you particularly liked?*

    Was there anything you particularly disliked?

26. *If mainstreamed at any point* – Did he/she have any specialist support? (Ask for all schools attended)

27. The general move these days is towards integrating deaf children. What do you think of this?

28. Was there a time when you felt particularly pleased about N's school experiences?

29. And a time when you felt unhappy?

30. At what age did he/she leave school?

31. Could you tell me if he/she got any certificates or qualifications at school?

	Preschool	Preschool/ school	School	School	School
Approx. age started					
Years spent there					
Age left					
Mainstream/special					
Communication					
School suggested/ parents chose					
Parents happy with school					
N happy with school					
What did you like most about it					
Exam passes/ certificates					

Could I ask you a little more about his/her last school?

32. What sort of things did the school do to prepare children for their lives after school?

    Probe   *Work experience?*

    Careers guidance?

    Life skills?

    Other?

33. Did N find this useful or do you feel that he/she needed more help than this? (Specify).

34. Did N have a clear idea about what he/she wanted to do after school?

   Probe *Had he/she always wanted to do this?*

   Do you feel that he/she was aiming too high or too low or did you feel that this was realistic?

   Did he/she ever want to do anything which you knew would not be possible because of his/her deafness?

35. Of all the people N has been involved with, who has done most to prepare him/her for his/her life after school?

36. Looking at the things he/she could do when he/she left school – What was N's reading like when he/she left school?

37. And what about now? What sort of things does he/she read now?

   Probe *Newspapers? (Specify)*

   Novels – fiction? (Specify)

   Non-fiction? (Specify)

   Magazines? (Specify)

   Ceefax/teletext?

38. Can you tell me of a situation which would pose difficulties for N's reading?

39. What about N's writing when he/she left school?

40. How would you describe it now?

41. Does he/she ever need to write these days?

   Probe *Letters/notes?*

   Forms?

   Poems?

   Essays?

42. Do you help him/her with his/her writing?

   Probe *In what ways?*

43. Can you describe a situation which would pose difficulties for N's writing?

44. At the end of school how was he/she able to cope with money?

45. And what about now?

   Probe   *Could you send him/her out to do some shopping for you?*

   Would he/she know if he/she had been given short change?

   Could you think of a situation which would cause N difficulties as far as money or numbers are concerned?

CURRENT SITUATION

46. Can you tell me first of all what N is doing now? Has he/she got a job or is he/she still training, or what?

   Probe   *Before his/her job did he/she go to college or university?*

47. Is he/she still living at home or has he/she left home?

   Probe   If full-time education elsewhere – *Is this still his/her home base in the holiday/vacations or does he/she have his/her own home now?*

48. Is he/she married or living with someone?

   Probe   If yes – *Have they any children?*

   Names and date of birth?

Move on to Part 2 according to whether N is:
A In a job – no full-time training (Pink)
B In a job – had full-time training (Green)
C In full-time training (Pale orange)
D Unemployed (Blue)
E At home with baby/children (Mauve)

Part 2

A IN A JOB – NO FULL-TIME TRAINING

49. Can you describe to me the job N actually does?

50. How long has he/she had the job?

> **Probe** *Who helped N in getting this job?*
>
> *Has he/she had other jobs? (Specify)*

51. Did he/she go straight from school into a job or was he/she unemployed for a time? (Specify in months)

52. *If appropriate* – How about between jobs? Has he/she been unemployed for any particular periods? (Specify in months, periods of unemployment)

53. Did he/she have any difficulty in finding jobs?

54. Has he/she done any training or further education since he/she left school?

55. Was the training for his/her job or attached to the job?

> **Probe** *Formal apprenticeship?*
>
> *Nightschool/day release?*
>
> *Other?*

56. Were any special arrangements made for N in this training?

> **Probe** *Support teacher?*
>
> *Extra time/attention?*
>
> *Seating?*
>
> *Other?*

57. What did he/she find most difficult about the training?

58. What did he/she enjoy most?

If unemployed at any time:

59. When N was unemployed did he/she seem troubled or did it not really bother him/her?

60. How did you feel about his/her situation?

61. How did he/she occupy him/herself during the day?

62. Were there times when you thought he/she'd never get another job?

63. How do you feel his/her deafness has influenced his/her job chances?

64. Do you feel that he/she is capable of more than he/she is actually doing?

    Probe   If yes – *In what ways?*

65. Do you feel that N is overstretched in his/her job?

66. Has/have his/her job(s) altered N as a person, do you think?

    Probe   *How?*

67. Does N seem clear about how his/her working life is going to be mapped out in the future or isn't he/she sure yet?

68. What do you think is most likely for him/her – how do you think things will develop for him/her so far as his/her work is concerned?

69. Is there anything which might get in the way of what he/she might achieve?

    Probe   *Deafness related?*

    Personality?

    Other?

B   IN A JOB – HAD FULL-TIME TRAINING

70. Can you describe to me the job N actually does?

71. Who helped N in getting this job?

72. Did N have any difficulty finding a job?

73. How long has he/she had the job?

    Probe   *Has he/she had other jobs? (Specify)*

74. Did he/she go straight from school into college or did he/she take any time off?

Probe *How long?*

Why?

What did he/she do in that time?

75. Could you tell me a little about his/her college life?

Probe *Special/mainstream?*

Support? (Specify)

Years spent there?

Any other deaf people (if mainstream)?

Age left?

Happy about it?

Greatest difficulty?

What liked most about it?

Qualifications/certificates?

76. Did he/she know what he/she wanted to do afterwards?

77. Did he/she go straight from college/university into a job or was he/she unemployed for a time? (Specify precisely)

Probe *How about between jobs? Has he/she been unemployed for any period? (Specify in months)*

If unemployed at any time:

78. When he/she was unemployed did he/she seem troubled or did it not really bother him/her?

79. How did you feel about his/her situation?

80. How did he/she occupy him/herself during the day?

81. Do you feel that N's deafness has influenced his/her job chances?

82. So, all in all, going back to N's job now, does he/she seem happy in this job or is he/she looking around for something better?

Probe *What kind of thing is he/she looking for?*

Is he/she hopeful of finding it?

Is this realistic?

83. Do you feel that he/she is capable of more than he/she is actually doing?

    Probe If yes – *In what ways?*

84. Is there (or has there been) any training attached to the job?

    Probe *Special arrangements?*

    Most difficult thing?

    Enjoyed most?

85. Do you feel that N is overstretched in his/her job?

    Probe *Is he/she understretched?*

86. Has N's job altered him/her as a person, do you think?

87. Does N seem clear about how his/her working life is going to be mapped out in the future, or isn't he/she sure yet?

88. What do you think is most likely for him/her – how do you think things will develop for him/her so far as work is concerned?

89. Is there anything which may get in the way of what he/she might achieve?

    Probe *Deafness related?*

    Personality?

    Other?

C IN FULL-TIME TRAINING

90. Can I get a few details about where N is studying?

    Probe *Name of institution?*

    Type of course? Full-time/sandwich?

    Entrance requirements of N?

    Name of course?

Length of course?

When did N start?

When will he/she finish?

Qualification at end?

91. Did N go straight from school to (name of institution), or what?

92. Could you tell me about the time between N's leaving school and starting (name of institution)?

      Probe   *Did he/she have any jobs?*

                Was he/she unemployed at any time?

If had jobs:

  Probe   *How long for?*

           Who helped N in getting this job?

           Any difficulty finding job(s)?

           Was he/she happy in the job or looking around for something better?

           Do you feel his/her deafness influenced his/her job chances?

           Did he/she do any training attached to the job?

           Special arrangements?

           Most difficult thing?

           Enjoyed most?

           Did you feel he/she was capable of more than he/she was actually doing?

           Overstretched/understretched?

           Did the job(s) alter him/her as a person, did you think?

If unemployed:

  Probe   *How long for?*

           When N was unemployed, did he/she seem troubled, or did it not really bother him/her?

           How did you feel about his/her situation?

How did he/she occupy him/herself during the day?

How do you feel that N's deafness has influenced his/her job chances?

93. Going back now to the course he/she is doing, could you tell me a little about his/her college life?

    Probe   *Special/mainstream?*

    Support? (Specify)

    Any other deaf people?

    Happy with it?

    Biggest problems/greatest difficulty?

    What liked most?

94. What does he/she want to do afterwards?

    Probe   *Is this realistic?*
    Will he/she need further training?

95. Do you feel that he/she is capable of more than he/she is actually doing?

    Probe   If yes – *in what ways?*

96. Do you feel that N is overstretched at college?

    Probe   *Is he/she understretched?*

97. Does N seem clear about how his/her working-life is going to be mapped out in the future or isn't he/she sure yet?

98. What do you think is most likely for him/her – how do you think things will develop for him/her so far as work is concerned?

99. Is there anything which might get in the way of what he/she might achieve?

    Probe   *Deafness related?*

    Personality?

    Others?

D UNEMPLOYED

100. Could you tell me a little about the time between N's leaving school and now?

> **Probe**   *Job?*
>
> *Training? (Full-time/part-time)*

If had a job:

101. Could you tell me a little about the jobs N has done? (Specify each)

> **Probe**   *Type of job?*
>
> *Any difficulties finding it?*
>
> *Who helped N to find it?*
>
> *Age?*
>
> *How long for?*
>
> *Why left?*

102. Did he/she go straight from school into a job, or what?

103. Was N happy in his/her job/in any of his/her jobs, or was he/she looking round for something better?

104. Did you feel that he/she was capable for more than he/she was actually doing?

> **Probe**   If yes – *In what ways?*

105. Did you feel that N was overstretched in his/her job?

> **Probe**   *Was he/she understretched?*

106. Did his/her job(s) alter him/her as a person, did you think?

107. What do you think has been his/her main problem with the jobs he/she's had?

108. What seems to be his/her main problem in getting a job now?

> **Probe** *Do you feel that his/her deafness has influenced his/her job chances?*

109. Did he/she think of going back to school/college to get any extra qualifications?

> **Probe** If yes – *How did that go?*
>
> If no – *What made him/her decide not to?*

If had training (not full-time)

110. You mentioned that he/she had some training – was this attached to his/her job?

> **Probe** *Formal apprenticeship?*
>
> *Night school/day release?*
>
> *Other?*

111. Were there any special arrangement for N?

> **Probe** *Support teacher?*
>
> *Extra attention?*
>
> *Seating?*
>
> *Other?*

112. What did he/she find most difficult about the training?

113. What did he/she enjoy most?

If had full-time training:

114. Did N. go straight from school into college, or did he/she take time off?

> **Probe** *How long?*
>
> *Why?*
>
> *What did he/she do in that time?*

115. Could you tell me a little about his/her college life?

> **Probe** *Special/mainstream?*
>
> *Support?*
>
> *Years spent there?*
>
> *Other deaf people? (If mainstream)*
>
> *Age left?*
>
> *Happy about it?*
>
> *Greatest difficulty?*
>
> *What he/she liked most about it?*
>
> *Qualifications/certificates?*
>
> *What did he/she want to do afterwards?*
>
> *What did he/she do afterwards?*
>
> *Did he/she go straight from college into a job, or what?*

Can I go back to talking about the present time?

116. How does N feel about being unemployed?

117. How do you feel about his/her situation?

118. How does N occupy him/herself during the day?

119. Are there times when either of you think he/she will never get a job/another job?

120. Does he/she seem to be looking for a job at the moment?

> **Probe** *What kind of thing is he/she looking for?*
>
> *Is this realistic, do you think?*
>
> *Is he/she hopeful of finding it?*

121. Does N seem to have any plans for his/her future as far as work is concerned?

122. How do you think things will develop for him/her as far as work is concerned?

123. Is there anything which might get in the way of what he/she might achieve?

>   Probe   *Deafness related?*
>
>   *Personality?*
>
>   *Other?*

E   AT HOME WITH BABY/CHILDREN

124. Could you tell me about the time between him/her leaving school and now?

125. What was he/she doing just prior to being at home with the baby?

>   Probe   *In job (no full-time training)? (A)*
>
>   *In job (had full-time training)? (B)*
>
>   *In full-time training? (C)*
>
>   *Unemployed? (D)*

Go to A/B/C/D and ask appropriately (i.e. past tense)

126. Do you think he/she will go back to work when *(name(s) of child/ children)* are older?

127. Do you think it may prove difficult to return?

>   Probe   *Why?*

Part 3

COMMUNICATION

I want to ask you about N's communication now. First of all, can we talk about the very early days when he/she first began to communicate?

128. When N was first diagnosed as deaf, did anyone advise you about the sort of communication you and he/she should use?

>   Probe   *Did you have any doubts or misgivings about this?*

129. Can you remember N's first word/sign?

>   **Probe** *How old was he/she when first said /used this?*

130. And what happened from then onwards? Did he/she chiefly use words, signs or gestures to communicate or a combination? *(Fill in table below)*

	Chiefly oral mode used with N	Chiefly gesture	Chiefly sign	Mixed specified
Parents				
Siblings				
Friends: deaf				
Friends: hearing				
Strangers				

Table indicates mode of communication used *by* N with others and by others *with* N.

131. Were you concerned about his/her communication in the early days?

If oral –

132. Were there any times when you felt you should introduce signing to him/her when he/she was younger?

133. Do you think he/she signed at school?

If signing –

134. Were there any times when you felt that you should have encouraged him/her to be more oral?

135. Did the school prefer an oral approach?

>   **Probe** *Did anyone ever discourage N from using signs?*

136. *If appropriate* – You say you use signs with N. When did you start to do this?

Probe *How did you learn?*

Did anyone encourage you, or was it your own decision?

137. When N was a child can you remember the sorts of situation which were particularly difficult for you to communicate about to him/her?

Probe *Something going to happen, e.g.*

Christmas/birthday/visits to school?

Could you give me an example?

138. And what about him/her? Can you think of times when he/she found it difficult to explain something to you?

139. When he/she was a child what was N's biggest problem in understanding other people?

140. And what were other people's biggest problems in understanding him/her?

141. Did you ever seek specialist help for N in his/her communication?

Probe *Specify?*

Why then?

Any help?

142. Looking back now, do you think anything could have been done to improve N's communication?

Probe *By you?*

By others?

143. Talking about communication **NOW**: How does he/she communicate now with...

	Chiefly oral	Chiefly gesture	Chiefly sign	Mixed specified	Mode used with N?
Parents					
Siblings					
Friends: deaf					

	Chiefly oral	Chiefly gesture	Chiefly sign	Mixed specified	Mode used with N?
Friends: hearing					
Strangers					

144. Can you tell me the particular **situations** which present difficulties for him/her in communicating with you now?

> **Probe**   *And what about with* strangers?

145. Can you tell me the sorts of **situations** which present difficulties for you in communicating with N now?

> **Probe**   *And what about strangers?*
>
> *What situations present difficulties for them in communicating with N?*

146. How well is he/she understood by...

	Very well	Quite well	Poorly
Parents			
Siblings			
Friends: deaf			
Friends: hearing			
Strangers			

147. And how well does he/she understand people?

	Very well	Quite well	Poorly
Parents			
Siblings			
Friends: deaf			
Friends: hearing			
Strangers			

148. Do you have difficulties in communicating about certain topics now?

    Probe   *Sexual matters (e.g. homosexuality)?*

              AIDS?

              Death?

              Other?

149. If N ever had an illness that meant he/she had to go to hospital, would it be difficult to explain it? (Would you have to stay with him/her?)

    Probe   *Has this ever happened in the past? Tell me about that.*

              Was communication a problem between N and staff/patients?

150. Has anyone close to N died or become seriously ill?

    Probe   *How did you explain this?*

              Were there any problems?

              Do you think N understood?

151. AIDS is a complicated disease for everyone to comprehend – do you think N understands about it or is he/she confused?

    Probe   If confused – *In what ways?*

              How have you tried to explain it?

              Has anyone else tried?

152. Young people these days seem to lead a more liberated life. Did you feel you had to explain the facts of life to N?

    Probe   *Did he/she understand?*

              Do you feel he/she is in any danger from the style of life he/she lives?

              Is there anything you felt you had to do about this?

              Have you ever worried that he/she was taking drugs/glue sniffing?

153. What about when he/she is unhappy – can he/she talk to you about this?

154. Has anything happened to you as a family which has been particularly difficult for N to comprehend and for you to explain?

155. Are there any things you've deliberately not told N because it was impossible/too difficult to explain?

156. Is there anything you thought he/she knew about but discovered some time later that he/she didn't?

157. Is it difficult to involve N in family decisions because he/she wouldn't understand?

   Probe   *Holidays?*

   Pet being put down?

   Moving house?

   Any other?

158. Has N experienced problems in situations in which he/she has to communicate with people outside the family?

   Probe   *Could you give me an example?*

   Work colleagues?

   Shop assistants?

   Doctor(s)?

   Talking with professional people generally (police, solicitors, social workers, etc.)?

   So does he/she take you or someone else with him/her? (Interpreters?)

159. Is there anything that he/she's understood that has surprised you?

160. Is there anything he/she's not understood that has surprised you?

161. Do you feel that because (sometimes) communication is a problem there are parts of his/her life you know nothing about?

   Probe   *Have you ever felt like this?*

162. Do you ever feel shut off from his/her life because communication is (sometimes) a problem?

   Probe   *Have you ever felt like this?*

163. Overall, how would you say N **feels** about his/her communication?

> Probe   *If we could ask him/her what do you feel he/she would say was the best/worst experience in his/her life as far as communication is concerned?*
>
> *Is that the best/worst for you, or would you describe another time?*

PERSONALITY AND EMOTION

164. Can you tell me a bit about N as a person now?

> Probe   *Calm/highly strung?*
>
> *Anxieties – does he/she have particular anxieties, like fear of heights or spiders?*
>
> *Bored/interested?*
>
> *Mood swings?*
>
> *Affectionate/reserved?*
>
> *Anything frightens him/her?*

165. Is he/she generally a happy or sad sort of person?

166. Is he/she bad-tempered or even-tempered?

> Probe   *Has he/she always been like this?*
>
> *Did he/she have a lot of temper tantrums as a child?*
>
> *When did these stop?*

167. Does he/she mind admitting he/she's in the wrong over something?

168. What are the main things that cause arguments between you?

> Probe   *Is it usually easy to resolve the arguments?*
>
> *Can you remember a particular incident when you fell out?*

169. Can N laugh at a joke about him/herself?

> Probe   *Does N ever tell jokes?*

FRIENDSHIPS/SOCIAL LIFE

What about N's friendships and social life:

170. When N was a child did he/she usually like to play alone or with other children?

     Probe *At primary school: alone/single others/group/special friend?*

     At secondary school: alone/single/group/special friend

171. Can you remember one special friend from his/her school days?

     Probe *How did they meet?*

     What did they do together?

     Could you describe their friendship?

     Are they still friends?

172. Has he/she kept in touch with friends from his/her school days or have they lost touch?

     Probe If yes – *How do they keep in touch?*

173. Did he/she ever find it difficult to make friends?

     Probe *Why do you feel this was so?*

     Did N seem to mind – was he/she ever lonely?

     Did he/she ever have imaginary friends?

174. Was there ever a time when you felt unhappy about any of his/her particular friends?

     Probe *Why was that?*

175. What about now: Is N a loner or does he/she have many friends?

     Probe If friends – *Friendship group/one single person/special friend?*

     Are they mostly male or female?

     How long have they been friends?

     If special – describe relationship

     How did he/she meet his/her friend/friends initially?

How does he/she make new friends **now***?*

What do they do together?

Where do they meet now?

Are you unhappy about any of his/her friends now?

If loner – *does he/she find it difficult to make friends?*

176. *If appropriate* – Has he/she made any friends at work?

      Probe *Do they meet out of work?*

177. Are his/her friends mostly deaf or hearing?

178. *If deaf* – When they talk together do you ever feel left out?

      Probe *Why?*

179. Is he/she a member of a deaf club?

      Probe If no – *Why do you think he/she has never joined?*

      If yes – *What do you think he/she gets out of that membership?*

If N is married/living with someone

180. Where did N meet ...?

181. Is ... deaf?

182. How long had they known each other before they lived together/got married?

183. Are you happy with the relationship, or was there ever a time when you felt concerned?

      Probe *Did you want N to marry a hearing person?*

      If deaf – *Did ...'s being deaf bother you?*

184. Do they seem to be getting along quite well, or would you say they have more than the average number of quarrels?

185. What are these usually about?

186. Are you optimistic about their marriage/relationship?

If children

187. How long were they together before they had their first child?

188. Is their child/are their children deaf?

If deaf **or** hearing

   Probe *What do you feel about this?*

If deaf

   Probe *Age of diagnosis?*

   Any early special tests?

   What was their reaction to the diagnosis?

   Were they advised about communication with (child's name)?

   What advice were they given?

   Did they take it?

   Were you happy about this?

   Is there any general advice you felt it important to give them?

189. N has a deaf/hearing mother and a deaf/hearing father. Do you feel that this causes him/her any difficulties at all?

190. How do you feel about the way ... is being brought up? Have you got any small worries?

191. Do you help them at all with the baby/children?

   Probe *Is this because they need help or just because you like to do it?*

192. Do you think that being a mother/father has changed N much?

MEDICAL

193. Can I look now at N's health: is he/she generally a healthy sort of person?

194. *If appropriate.* You said that N is easily depressed. Has it ever been necessary for him/her to take tranquillisers or anti-depressant tablets in the past to help with this?

Probe   *Is he/she still taking them?*

Did he/she spend any time in hospital for this?

195. When he/she was a child you said...about his/her sleeping.

    Probe   *Is sleeping still a problem for him/her?*

    When did these early difficulties end?

196. Has he/she had any lengthy treatment associated with his/her deafness?

    Probe   *Lourdes?*

    Cochlear implant?

    Faith healers?

    Alternative medicine?

    Other?

197. What about the future – are you/is he/she planning any treatment?

198. Has N ever had any serious illnesses?

Age	Length of illness	Specify	Treatment

199. Has N ever been involved in an accident?

    Probe   *Could you tell me a little about this?*

CONFLICT AND DANGER

200. Does N do anything that worries you because it is dangerous?

201. What about the places he/she goes to? Is he/she ever in danger of finding him/herself in a situation he/she can't handle?

    Probe   *Has N ever got into any real fights or violence, as far as you know?*

    Has he/she ever got into trouble because of a misunderstanding?

202. Has he/she ever got into trouble with the police?

> **Probe** *What about?*
>
> *Was he/she charged?*
>
> *Do you think his/her deafness caused any problems in giving explanations?*
>
> *Were any special arrangements made to help him/her explain his/her side of the story?*
>
> *Are you worried about N getting into trouble again?*

INDEPENDENCE

203. As a child you said (give details). What about now? Would you say that N is a very independent person?

> **Probe** *Can he/she read and follow a bus timetable?*
>
> *Can he/she drive? Will he/she drive on his/her own? How far?*
>
> *Will he/she use public transport alone? (bus/plane/train)*
>
> *Does he/she go shopping on his/her own?*
>
> *Does he/she go to the doctor's alone?*
>
> *Does he/she handle his/her own finances, or do you have to help him/her out?*
>
> *Has he/she got a bank account?*
>
> *Has he/she got a credit card?*
>
> *Has he/she a home of his/her own and can he/she cope?*

204. Obviously, N's legally grown up now, but are there any ways in which he/she still seems like a child/immature to you?

If living at home

205. N is still living at home – do you feel that this is a good or a bad thing on the whole?

206. Would you normally expect a person of this age to be living at home?

207. Are there any problems which arise directly out of the fact that he/she's still at home?

208. Are there any advantages?

If left home

209. How did his/her leaving home come about? Was it a sudden decision or did it happen gradually?

    Probe *Was there a particular reason for it?*

210. How did you feel at the time – were you happy for him/her to go?

    Probe *Do you have any worries about him/her living away from home?*

If left home/at college

211. How closely are you in touch when he/she's away?

    Probe *How often do you see him/her?*

212. How do you keep in touch?

    Probe *Is it usually you who calls/writes?*

    If you needed to get a message to him/her urgently, how would you do it?

EFFECTS OF DEAFNESS ON FAMILY AND SIBLINGS

213. How does N get on with his/her brothers and sisters?

214. Would you say that in the past any of his/her brothers and sisters have resented N?

    Probe *Why do you feel this was so?*

    Did they lose friends because of him/her?

215. What about now? Do any of his/her brothers and sisters resent N?

    Probe *Why do you feel this is so?*

216. Even if there is no resentment, it is sometimes difficult being the brother/ sister of a deaf person. Can you think of a time when this was so when N was a child?

     Probe *Did they lose friends because of him/her?*

217. Do you think that they have a sense of future responsibility for N?

     Probe *Is it likely that he/she might live with one of them later on in life?*

     Have you made any particular arrangements for N later on?

218. The pressures of bringing up a child with a handicap can sometimes put pressure on family relationships in general. Were there times when you felt that your family life was under strain?

     Probe How?

     What about you and your husband/wife – did bringing up N cause difficulties for you as a couple?

219. Do you feel that your health or the health of anyone in the family suffered due to the effects of N's deafness?

     Probe *Did your social life suffer?*

     Did you miss holidays because of N?

     Did either your own or your partner/husband's work suffer?

220. Talking generally now – in what ways has your family life been different from what might have been if N had not been deaf?

     Probe *Has N's presence ever made family life difficult?*

     What about for other members of the family. Are they quite comfortable with N (embarrassment)?

REFLECTIONS

221. Would you say that there was a time when he/she realised that he/she was deaf and so different from hearing people?

     Probe *When was this?*

     What happened?

Did he/she seem sad or angry in any way?

What about now? Does he/she seem bitter?

Either

222. You did not have any more children. Was this because of the risk of deafness?

     Or

223. You went on to have more children. Did you feel that there might be any risk of having more deaf children?

224. If you had to advise the parents of a newly diagnosed deaf child, is there anything you feel would be a very important thing to say?

     Probe   *Who would you advise them to go to for help?*

     Have you ever found it useful to contact other parents of deaf children? (What about now?)

225. Was there any bad advice you were given.

     Probe   *Or advice you felt was insensitive/misinformed/harmful?*

     Did you feel you had too much advice or too little?

226. Has anybody been particularly helpful to you?

     Probe   *Social Worker?*

     Teacher of Deaf?

     Chaplain?

     Family friend?

     Doctor?

     Other?

227. Overall, what do you feel is the most important change N's deafness has made to your life?

228. What was the best time you've had together?

229. What was the most difficult time?

230. If N had been born now, do you think his/her life would have been very different?

> **Probe** *What about his/her education?*
>
> *Integration?*
>
> *Use of language?*

231. Do you think that attitudes to deafness have changed over the last 20 years?

> **Probe** *How?*
>
> *If not – why not?*

232. Looking to the future now, do you have any particular worries?

233. What do you hope for N in the future?

DEAF YOUNG PEOPLE'S SCHEDULE

Date of interview   Interviewer
N's name and address
Tel
Date of Birth
Age

Guidelines for interviewer

(1) Before interview make clear:
   (a) The purpose of the interview;
   (b) That the interview will be confidential;
   (c) That some of the questions are personal and the interviewee is free to decide not to answer them.

(2) As far as possible ask all the questions in roman type. Those in italics are to be used as probes at your discretion.

(3) In some cases questions will have to be omitted because they are inappropriate or the interviewee will not understand them. In some cases questions may have to be elaborated and expanded to get an answer. All these

circumstances should be discussed with the notetaker afterwards so that they can be appropriately coded.

(4) In extreme cases the interviewee may have difficulty in understanding the questions and the schedule will have to be abandoned. In this case general questions should be put on the topics specified in heavy type.

Guidelines for notetaker

(1) All answers given should be taken down as fully as possible.

(2) Question omitted should be marked '0'. After the interview discuss with the interviewer why questions were omitted. Those that were inappropriate or not applicable should be marked 'ONA', those that it was felt would not be understood by the interviewee should be marked 'ONU'.

(3) If the interviewee does not answer a question that has been put, it should be marked 'NA' if he/she indicates it is not applicable, and 'NU' if he/she indicates it is not understood.

(4) Any question which the interviewer elaborates or expands upon in detail, should be starred, and the answer recorded.

(5) If the interviewee abandons the schedule, take as full notes as possible under the relevant section headings.

Key

ONA	Omitted not applicable
ONU	Omitted not understood
NA	Asked but not applicable
NU	Asked but not understood
*	Question answered after elaboration and explanation by interviewer

---

DEAFNESS

1. Do you know what your hearing loss is?

2. Do you know why you are deaf?

3. What kind of hearing aid(s) have you got? (ask to see if appropriate)

   If aids – *How often do you wear it/them?*

   Can you tell me how helpful it is to wear hearing aids?

   Should deaf children be made to wear hearing aids?

4. What can you hear?

> **Probe** *Machinery working?*
>
> *Someone shouting?*
>
> *Baby crying?*
>
> *Dog barking?*
>
> *Telephone ringing?*

5. What can you do?

> **Probe** *Follow a person talking by lip reading and listening?*
>
> *Tell whether it is a man or a woman on the 'phone?*
>
> *Use the 'phone in code?*
>
> *Understand someone close on the 'phone?*
>
> *Understand anyone on the 'phone (if they know you are deaf)?*
>
> *Follow rhythm?*
>
> *Recognise a tune?*
>
> *Play a musical instrument?*
>
> *Play music and recognise if a note is wrong?*

PREPARATION FOR LEAVING SCHOOL AND POST-SCHOOL EXPERIENCE

This section of the interview should ask the interviewee to talk about their life, in chronological order, starting with their preparation for leaving school. It should be as free a conversation as possible, following up issues as seems appropriate.

However, the coloured sheets give a list of questions that should be asked as and when relevant. Questions should be changed to refer to past situations as appropriate. These are as follows:

A. Preparation for work   Sun yellow sheet
B. Job interviews   Lime green sheet
C. Work   Pink sheet
D. Training   Pale orange sheet
E. Unemployment   Blue Sheet
F. If has baby/child   Mauve sheet

Note: The colours correspond with the interview schedule for the parents, but not the letters.

(This section should not take more than half an hour.)

Preparation for work

A.1. Before you left school did you do any voluntary work, paid work or get any work experience?

A.2. *Either*

What did you do?

> **Probe**   *Did it help you learn to get on with people?*
>
> *Did it help you decide what you wanted to do – or what you did not want to do?*
>
> *Did it help you get a job?*
>
> *Would you have liked more or less work experience?*
>
> *Why?*

Or

Can you tell me why you did not get any experiences of working?

> **Probe**   *Never thought of it?*
>
> *School did not encourage?*
>
> *Parents never thought?*
>
> *Parents did not encourage?*
>
> *Not had opportunity?*
>
> *Brothers and sisters did not, therefore not expected in family?*
>
> *Health reasons?*
>
> *Other?*

Do you wish you had had the appropriate work experience?
If yes – Why?

A.3. At school did you have group discussions about work and relationships at work?

Probe *Did you role play interviews?*

A.4. Before you left school did you get any support or information about careers or getting a job?

> *If yes:* What information?
>   Who from?

Probe *Careers guidance?*

Teachers of the Deaf?

Family/friends/contacts?

A.5. Now I am going to ask you a 'just suppose' question.

If you had a deaf child/teenager coming up to leaving school, would you encourage him/her to get some experience of working?

Probe *Would you have liked this for yourself?*

Job interviews

B.1. Tell me what happened on your last interview for a job.

> **Probe** *How did you hear about the job??*
>
> *Did you get the application form yourself and did you complete it yourself?*
>
> *Did you arrange transport yourself to get to the place of interview?*
>
> *Did you go into the interview yourself or with another person?*
>
> *Did another person interpret, speak for you or what?*
>
> *Did you tell interviewer/or on application form that you are deaf?*
>
> *Did you stop the interview when you didn't understand?*

Work

C.1. Tell me about the job you have now.

C.2. Did you have difficulty in finding a job?

> *If yes* – Was it a problem finding a job you liked or just finding one at all?

C.3. Are you happy in this job?

> *If not happy in job*
>
>> **Probe** *What is the main problem with this job?*
>>
>>   *Are you looking for another job that suits you better?*
>>
>>   If yes – *What kind of thing are you looking for?*
>>
>>   *Are you hopeful that you will find what you want?*

C.4. Is there any training attached to this job?

> *If yes* – What sort of training is it?
>
> *If no* – Would you like to have training?
>
> *If yes* – What? Is it possible for you to study this?

C.5. Are you quite clear about how your working life is going to be in the future or are you not sure?

>> **Probe** How would you like things to develop at work?
>>
>>   What is there that might stop you achieving what you want?

Training

D.1. Have you ever had any training for work?

> *If yes* – How long is the training course(s)?
>
>   How far have you got with your course(s)?
>
>   What certificate do you hope to get at the end of the course(s)?

D.2. Are you getting any specialist help because of your deafness?

>> **Probe** *Teacher of the deaf?*
>>
>>   *Radio aid?*
>>
>>   *Lip speaker?*
>>
>>   *Interpreter?*
>>
>>   *Extra tuition?*
>>
>>   *Notetakers?*

D.3. How do you get on with other students on the course?

> **Probe** *Are the students helpful and friendly or not?*
>
> *Do you get on with a few students or most of the students?*
>
> *Why do you feel this is?*
>
> *What is communication like between you and the students?*
>
> *Can you understand most of the students?*
>
> *Are most of the students able to understand you?*
>
> *Do you socialise with the students?*

If yes – *What sort of things do you do together?*

D.4. What are the tutors like?

> **Probe** *Are some tutors better than others?*
>
> If yes – *How?*
>
> *Are there any difficult or bad tutors?*
>
> If yes – *How?*

D.5. Were you ready for the course?

> **Probe** *Could you have done with pre-course training?*
>
> *Do you feel you were on the same level as the other students?*
>
> *What would you recommend to any deaf student going on a course or to study generally?*

D.6. Either

Do you think you will complete the course successfully?

Or

Did you complete the course successfully?
If no – Why not?

Unemployed

E.1. I understand you have not got a job. Can you explain why you are not working?

> **Probe** *No jobs available?*

Refused training?

No opportunity for jobs to particular liking?

Family commitment?

Out of choice?

Illness physical/mental?

Disliked Government training schemes?

Too low pay?

Personality clashes?

Disliked idea of working away?

Sacked?

Redundant?

Never worked?

No suitable jobs with my qualifications?

E.2. Are you looking for work?

   If no – Have you given up?

   If yes – How are you looking for work?

   Probe   *Job Centre?*

   Job Shop?

   UB40 Club?

   Private employment agencies?

   Magazines?

   Newspapers?

   Library?

   Teletext?

E.3. Have you had any help in looking for work?

   Probe   *Disablement Resettlement Officer?*

   Social Worker with Deaf People?

   Teacher of the Deaf?

Disability Advisory Service?

School?

Voluntary organization?

Internal – friends/relations/partner?

Specialist careers advisers?

E.4. If you could create your own job, what would you like to do?

If has baby/child

F.1. Did having a baby/child make any difference to your feelings about your job/training?

    Probe *Has it made things difficult for you in any way?*

F.2. Is your girl/boyfriend (wife/husband) working or in full-time training?

    Part-time/full-time/home-work/training ...time/name.

F.3. Do you feel your partner is doing as much for the baby/child(ren) as you are or does he/she expect you to take the main responsibility for looking after them/him/her?

F.4. Some people think it is a good idea for the mother to go out to work and the father to look after the children. Have you ever considered that?

    Probe *What would your partner feel about that?*

PERSONALITY AND EMOTION

6. Can you tell me what kind of a person you are?

    Probe *Happy/sad?*

            Calm/get easily worked up?

            Creative – thinks of ideas/not good at creative thinking?

            Easily trust people/don't find it easy to trust people?

            Confident/not very confident?

            Show your feelings/keep feelings to yourself?

7. Is there anything that makes you anxious?

> **Probe**   *Fear of heights?*
>
> *Spiders?*
>
> *Others?*

8. Is there anything you avoid doing because it makes you anxious?

> **Probe**   *Groups of people?*

9. Do you like yourself?

> **Probe**   *Do you ever feel proud of yourself? (Examples)*
>
> *Do you ever feel sorry for yourself? (Examples)*

10. Is there anything about yourself you do not like and want to change?

11. Is there anyone you admire and would like to be similar to?

COMMUNICATION

Communication and family life

12. How well do you understand your family?

> **Probe**   *Parents?*
>
> *Siblings?*
>
> *Spouse/partner/boy or girlfriend?*
>
> *(Specify usual mode of communication: speech, signing, gesture, mixed)*

13. How well do other people understand you?

> **Probe**   *Parents?*
>
> *Siblings?*
>
> *Spouse/partner boy or girlfriend?*
>
> *(Specify usual mode of communication: speech, signing, gesture, mixed)*
>
> *If siblings*

14. Did your brother(s) and/or sister(s) ever interpret/speak/listen for you?

> **Probe** *Did they ever tell you what your parents wanted you to do?*
>
> If yes – *What did you feel about that?*

15. Do you remember times in the past when your family got together and talked?

> **Probe** *Mealtimes?*
>
> *Special occasions, e.g. Christmas?*
>
> If yes – *How did you feel about it?*
>
> *Could you follow the conversation?*

16. What happens at family gatherings now?

> **Probe** *Could your family improve their communication with you?*
>
> If yes. – *In what way?*

17. Were your mother and father able to explain to you about things that were going to happen?

> **Probe** *Christmas?*
>
> *Birthdays?*
>
> *Visits and outings?*
>
> *Starting school?*
>
> *Changing school*

18. Did your mother and father discuss personal matters with you?

> **Probe** *Friendships?*
>
> *Sexual behaviour?*
>
> *Death?*

19. Were you included in decisions that were made in the family?

> **Probe** *Holidays?*
>
> *Pets being put down?*
>
> *Moving house?*

20. Some deaf people have said that something important happened with their families and they did not find out until later. Did that happen to you?

   Probe   *Death in the family?*

   Illness in the family?

   Other family members moved house?

21. Have you ever found out that your parents lied to you?

   If yes – *Can you tell me about that?*

   Do you understand why they lied?

22. Were there ever difficult times at home? (Specify)

23. Was it ever difficult to explain something to your mother and father?

   Probe   *Were you ever surprised at something they understood?*

24. There must have been times when you were unhappy or in trouble. Was there anyone in the family you would go to then?

   Probe   *Parents?*

   Brother(s)/sister(s)?

   Grandparents?

   Other?

25. Do you have the opportunity to talk things over in depth with your family?

   If yes – *Give details?*

26. Can you tell me about particularly happy times you remember with your family?

27. Were you treated differently by your family because you were deaf?

   Probe   *More lenient/stricter? (Examples)*

   Overprotected/pushed too hard? (Examples)

   Low expections/high expectations? (Examples)

If siblings

28. Did you go around with your brother(s) and/or sister(s)?

> **Probe** *Were they jealous of you?*
>
> If yes – *Why?*
>
> *Were you jealous of them?*
>
> If yes – *Why?*

29. Do you think any of your family suffered because you are deaf?

> **Probe** *Relationship with family?*
>
> *Family member problems at home/school/with police?*
>
> *Additional stress/mental illness?*

30. *If appropriate*

Do you think life has been better for any of your family because you are deaf?

31. Has one of your parents ever 'walked out' for a period of time?

> If yes – *Can you tell me about it?*
>
> *Did you know about it at the time?*
>
> *What did you feel about it when you found out?*

> *If parents separated or divorced*

32a. Were you aware that your parents' relationship was breaking down?

32b. How did you feel at the time they split up?

> **Probe** *Want to blame someone?*
>
> *Want them to get back together?*
>
> *Betrayed?*
>
> *Disappointed?*
>
> *Relieved?*
>
> *Happier?*

33. *If living away from home*

You are not living at home now. How did it happen – was it a sudden decision or did it happen gradually?

Probe   *Was there a particular reason for it?*

How did you feel at the time?

How did your parents feel at the time – were they happy to let you go?

What things worried them?

If living at home

You live at home at the moment. Have you thought about leaving home?

Probe   *When do you think this will be?*

What could make you leave home?

34. How often do you see/hear from them now that you are living away from home?

Probe   *How do you keep in touch?*

Is it mostly you who calls/writes to your parents, or mostly them?

If you need to get a message to them urgently how would you do it?

How would they contact you in an emergency?

Communication – general

35. I would like to ask you now about how you communicate with people in general, and how they communicate with you.

(Establish for three or four of the following as appropriate)

Doctor

Chaplain (general)

Chaplain with the deaf

Social worker (general)

Social worker with the deaf

Sign language interpreter

    Police

    Public transport personnel

    DHSS personnel

    Driving instructor

    Lawyer

    (Specify: speech, gesture, sign language, written notes, lip speaking, interpreting, combination)

36. What would you feel now if someone close to you corrects your speech?

37. Do you think your speech has improved or not since leaving school?

38. How do you manage in following conversations with a group of hearing friends?

    Probe   *At work?*

              In a pub?

39. Do you get angry or hurt when hearing people talk and you do not undertand what they are saying?

    If yes – *What do you do about this?*

40. Do you ever feel hearing people are talking about you?

    If yes – *What sort of situations?*

Sign language

41. Do you remember where and when you first saw sign language being used?

    If yes – Do you remember how you felt at the time?

    Probe   *Curious?*

              Interested?

              Attracted?

              Embarrassed?

              Shocked?

              Repulsed?

42. At that time what had you been told about sign language?

   Probe *Proper language/ not a language?*

   Helps speech/does not help speech?

   Helps lip reading/does not help lip reading?

43. Do you think speaking deaf people are cleverer than signing deaf people?

   If yes – *Why?*

44. What do your parents think about sign language?

   Probe *Have they always felt this?*

45. Were you allowed to use sign language or finger spelling when you were younger?

	Forbidden	Discouraged	Allowed	Encouraged
In class				
In playground				
At home				
At Deaf Club				

   If forbidden or discouraged

   Probe *What happened if you were caught using sign language/finger spelling/no voice?*

   If not already answered

46. Can anyone close to you use sign language?

   Probe *Has anyone close to you tried to learn/thought of learning sign language?*

47. Do you know of any television programmes that use sign language?

   If yes – *Has it changed your views about sign language?*

48. Now I am going to ask a 'just suppose' question.

   If you had a very deaf child how would you communicate with him or her?

SCHOOLING

49. Which schools did you go to?

50. *Either*

At which school were you happiest and why?

Or

In which part of the school were you happiest and why?

Probe *Educational aspects?*

Social aspects?

51. What of the things you did at school were most useful to you?

Probe *Help in deciding about a career?*

Management and running a home?

Developing self confidence and independence?

Education in the practical aspects of everyday life?

Training in decision making?

52. Was anything you did at school a waste of time?

53. When you were at school what technical aids did you use?

Probe *Hearing aids?*

Radios or phonic aids?

Loop?

Auditory trainer?

Other?

Speech trainer? (group or 1:1)

54. What did you find the most helpful?

Probe *Was there anything that was not helpful?*

55a. Do you feel your school expected too much of you?

Probe *Did they expect too little?*

55b. How did you feel when you first left school?

FRIENDSHIP

School friends

56. What about friends at school: Did you have any special friends?

57. *If special friends* – Were they the same age as you or younger or older?

Were they deaf or hearing?

58. *Either*

Who did you see outside school hours?

   Probe   *School friends?*

Neighbours?

None?

Or

Who did you see at weekends or holidays?

   Probe   *School friends?*

Neighbours?

None?

59. When you were at school were you involved in any clubs or groups?

   If yes – Were these deaf or hearing groups?

Who encouraged you to join?

   If no – Were you aware of clubs or groups for deaf and/or hearing people in your area?

60. Did your parents disapprove of any of your school friends?

   If yes – Can you tell me about this?

61. Can you tell me about some of the good times you had with your school friends?

62. What do you feel abour your school friends now – do you keep in contact?

   If yes – How?

63. Do you think your parents could have helped you more in making friends when you were young?

    If yes – In what way?

64. Did you know that some young hearing children have imaginary friends? Can you remember if you had any imaginary friends?

    If yes – Can you tell me about it?

65. Now I am going to ask you a rather difficult question – if you had a school-age deaf child, how would you give your child the opportunity to make friends?

    Probe   *Would you have liked this for yourself?*

Friendship now

What about your friends now?

66. Have you any close friends?

    If yes – What ages?

    What jobs do they do?

    Are they deaf or hearing?

    How often do you see each other?

    What do you do together?

    If no – Can you explain why you have no close friends?

67. Do you spend time on your own?

    If yes – What do you do?

Boyfriends/girlfriends/partners

Now I am going to ask you some rather personal questions – let me remind you that you should not feel you have to answer them.

68. *Either*

    Have you a boyfriend/girlfriend now?

    Or

You are married/living with someone/have a permanent girlfriend/boyfriend.

If never had boyfriend/girlfriend go to 76

69. Is your husband/wife/partner/boyfriend/girlfriend deaf or hearing?

    Probe   *Do you think deaf people should have deaf/hearing partners?*

70. Do you feel this is a good relationship for you?

    Probe   *In what way does he/she make your life better?*

    In what way do you make life better for him/her?

71. What do your parents feel about your relationship?

72. Before you left school did you have boy friends/girl friends?

    If yes – Some people have boy friends/girl friends because it is expected of them. Was it like this for you?

73. *Either*

    What is your ideal partner – deaf or hearing?

    Or

    Before you met ... did you feel your ideal partner would be deaf or hearing?

Sexual behaviour

74. How did you learn about sex?

    Probe   *Family?*

    School teachers?

    Classmates?

    Books?

    Trial and error?

    Other

75. In looking back who do you think should have the responsibility of telling you about sex and relationships?

76. If you have problems with your relationship or with sex who would you go to talk about it?

77. Do you want children?

> **Probe** *Deaf children?*
>
> *Hearing children?*

CURRENT AFFAIRS AND SOCIAL ISSUES

AIDS

78. Do you know about the dangers of AIDS?

> *If yes* – How did you know about it?
>
> What do you feel about people who have AIDS?

Drugs

79. Has anyone talked to you about drugs and glue sniffing?

80. Have you ever been in company of those who have used drugs?

> *If yes* – Have you seen what happens to them?

81. Have you ever experimented with drugs?

> **Probe** *Has there been a situation where someone has offered you drugs without you knowing they were drugs?*

Politics and religion

82. Does your family ever talk about politics?

> **Probe** If yes – *Do you join in?*

83. Did you vote in the last election?

> *If no* – Why not?
>
> *If yes* – How did you vote?
>
> Is this because of family vote or because it was your own decision?

84. Do you go to Church?

    Probe *Do you talk about God?*

85. I would like to ask your opinion on some matters.

    A. Margaret Thatcher is a good Prime Minister.

    Yes/No/Complex/Don't know

    B. Neil Kinnock could be a better Prime Minister.

    Yes/No/Complex/Don't know

    C. Nuclear power is safe to make.

    Yes/No/Complex/Don't know

    D. Black people should rule South Africa.

    Yes/No/Complex/Don't know

    E. Women should not go to work but stay at home.

    Yes/No/Complex/Don't know

    F. All policemen should have guns.

    Yes/No/Complex/Don't know

    G. Violence on TV makes violence in real life worse.

    Yes/No/Complex/Don't know

    H. It is bad for couples to live together without getting married.

    Yes/No/Complex/Don't know

    I. The British Army should come out of Ireland.

    Yes/No/Complex/Don't know

    J. Most people who are out of work are too lazy to look for work.

    Yes/No/Complex/Don't know

    K. Rape is a serious crime.

    Yes/No/Complex/Don't know

    L. Abortion is a woman's decision.

    Yes/No/Complex/Don't know

    M. Hanging should be brought back.

    Yes/No/Complex/Don't know

N. It is all right for gay people to live together.

Yes/No/complex/Don't know

Newspapers, books and television

86. Do you read a newspaper?

   Probe *Every day/sometimes/rarely/never*

87. Which newspaper is the one you read most recently?

   Probe *Daily Mirror (local)*

   Daily Express

   Guardian

   Sun

   Daily Mail

   Times

   Today

   Star

   Telegraph

   Evening paper

   Local daily

   News of the World

88. Which part of the paper do you read?

   Probe *Political news?*

   Financial news?

   News about everyday things?

   Sports news?

   Just whatever looks interesting?

89. Do you read magazines?

   Probe *Women's?*

   Hobby?

> *Special interest?*
>
> *British Deaf News?*
>
> *Comic?*
>
> *Teenager magazine?*
>
> *Car?*
>
> *Sports?*
>
> *Journal?*

90. Do you read books?

    Every day/regularly/sometimes/ very rarely/never

91. What was the last book you read?

    > *Romance?*
    >
    > *Spy?*
    >
    > *Science fiction?*
    >
    > *Thriller?*
    >
    > *History?*
    >
    > *Other?*
    >
    > *Non-fiction?*
    >
    > *Can't remember?*

92. Do you watch television?

    Probe *What programmes?*

    Have you teletext?

    If yes – *Which programmes would you like to see subtitled that are not already?*

93. What technological aids have helped you most?

    Probe *Teletext?*

    Visual telecommunication system, i.e. Vistel?

    Hearing aids?

> *Radio aids?*
>
> *Flashing door bell?*
>
> *Other?*

POLITICS OF DEAFNESS

94. What would you like the government to do for deaf people?

     Probe *Do you know of anything the government has recently (last 10 years) done for deaf people?*

95. Would you like to have a sign language interpreter on news programmes?

96. Do you think there should be a news programme run and presented by deaf people themselves?

97. Do you think deaf people need to get involved with Councillors and MPs to get some changes to improve things for deaf children and adults?

     If yes – Do you think deaf people can do this?

     Probe *How?*

98. Do you think the deaf programmes like See Hear or Listening Eye are helpful in educating the public about deaf people?

99. Are you involved in any Deaf organisation?

     Probe *British Deaf Association*

     National Deaf Children's Society

     Royal National Institute for the Deaf

     British Association of the Hard of Hearing

     Deaf Broadcasting Council

100. Is there any Deaf Club/group you have been to which you feel is really good?

     Why is this?

REFLECTIONS

This is the last section and I would like to ask you to look back on your life and think about the future.

101. How would life be different if you were not deaf?

102. How old were you when you first became aware that you were different?

    Probe   *Can you tell me about it?*

103. Some deaf children think that one day they might be hearing. Did you ever think that?

    Probe   *Do you know if any of your deaf friends ever thought this?*

104. Has there ever been a time when you wished you were hearing?

    If yes – Do you now? (Specify)

105. In your dreams are you deaf or hearing?

    Probe   *How do you communicate with others, and others with you in your dreams?*

106. Do you think life is different for deaf children born today?

107. Do you have any views on how deaf children should be educated?

    Probe   *Integration?*

    Use of sign language in schools?

108. Do you think deaf children in Units and mainstream schools today will go on to join Deaf Clubs?

109. Have you any worries about the future?

110. What do you most look forward to in the future?

Demographic information

Of the 101 families that were sought, 91 were traced and 83 interviewed (Table A.1). With the 82 parents interviewed, 71 of the young people were interviewed (Table A.2). Of the 71 young people interviewed, 61 interviews were used in the quantitative analysis (Table A.3). The parents who were interviewed are shown in Table A.4.

Most of the interviews were carried out by Juliet Bishop, with just two by Susan Gregory. In 47 (57%) of the parent interviews, the young person was not present; in 16 (20%) they were there for part of the time and in 19 (23%) there for all the time. Only ten families had moved away from the East Midlands since the first interview, though of course it is likely that a higher number of those in the non-contact group had moved away.

In the following tables (Tables A.5–A.9) information from the parents' sample of interviews (82) is given first, followed by that from the young people's sample (61).

Table A.1. *Families in study*

	Number
Parents interviewed	83 (82)*
Not traced	10
Deafness not main issue	3 (4)*
Young person not deaf	2
Family emigrated	1
Young person died	1
Father of young person seriously ill	1

Note: one of these interviews was not used in the analysis as deafness was not the main issue. Final figures: parents interviewed, 82; deafness not the main issue, 4.

Table A.2. *Reasons for not interviewing 11 of the young people*

	Number
Parents suggest that young person's communication skills not adequate for interview	4
Young person refused or failed to respond to attempts to arrange an interview	6
Parents refused on behalf of the young person	1

Table A.3. *Reasons for not using ten of the interviews*

	Number
Young person visited, interview not attempted	1
Young person visited, interview abandoned	3
Young person interviewed, interview not coded	2
Young person interviewed, interview coded, but not used*	4

Note: *The interview was not used when 20% or more of the responses could not be coded.

Table A.4. *Who was interviewed in the parents' interviews*

	Number
One person	
Mother	35
Father	1
Stepmother	1
Sister	1
Foster mother	1
Total	39
Two people	
Mother and father	35
Mother and stepfather	6
Stepmother and father	1
Stepmother and stepfather	1
Total	43

Note: In all quote descriptions, for convenience and to protect confidentiality, these are described as mother or father, unless it is necessary to be more specific.

Table A.5. *Sex of sample*

	Parents	Young people
Female	34	28
Male	48	33

Table A.6. *Age of sample at time of parent interview*

Age (years)	Parents	Young people
18	3	3
19	13	9
20	18	14
21	22	15
22	18	13
23	4	3
24	4	4

Table A.7. *Preferred communication of young people*

	Parents	Young people
BSL	31	24
SSE	13	11
Oral	30	26
LLS	8	0

Table A.8. *Functional hearing loss based on information from parent interview*

	Parents	Young people
Profound loss	31	18
Severe loss	30	25
Moderate loss	13	10
Partially hearing	8	8

Table A.9. *Disabilities of the deaf young people specified by parents*

	Parents	Young people
Learning difficulties	6	0
Physical disability	4	3
Visual impairment	2	0
Autism	1	1
Heart problems	1	1
Multiple (physical/heart)	1	1
Apraxia	1	1

APPENDIX III

Interviewing deaf young people and their families

THE INTERVIEW AS A RESEARCH TOOL

I am saying this as much for you as for us

This book is based on interviews with parents in the early 1970s and with parents and deaf young people in the late 1980s. In carrying out the research we have been interested in the way in which the understanding of the interview process and accounts of responses to interviews has undergone changes in this period.

In the early 1970s, the main concern in devising the interview schedules was how to get people to tell the 'truth' and how to check that the answers were truthful. In this process, attention was paid to both the perceived status of the interviewer and the interview questions themselves. Newson & Newson, whose work was a precursor to the research reported here, describe how the shift from health visitor to university interviewer resulted in a change in responses to particular questions (e.g. concerning the use of dummies) from the parents interviewed in their study (1963). In their research, as in the first set of interviews that form the basis of this book, questions were carefully constructed to get at the 'truth'. For example, in the questions about bed wetting in four year olds, who might be expected to be dry at night, the preamble to the set of questions was, 'I expect he (sic) still wets the bed sometimes doesn't he?' to make it as easy as possible to give the socially less desirable response. Other techniques used were to probe the same topic in a number of different ways (Newson & Newson, 1963, 1968).

However, more recently, the emphasis in interview-based research has been on the ways in which people account for their own lives and experience. In constructing and using the later interviews, our intention was to ask those questions that would allow interviewees to tell us about their lives and experiences in ways that were appropriate for them. Their responses were conceived, not in terms of truth or falsehood, but as ways of accounting for, or explaining, their particular experience. Such an approach could apply to any interview-based research; however, we feel it to be particularly significant for parents talking about their deaf sons or daughters. These parents did not expect to have a deaf child, and initially, at least, were unlikely to know anyone in the same position. For most people, child rearing takes place in the context of knowledge held in common with relations or friends, with an established 'taken for granted' set of expectations and behaviours. With a deaf son or daughter, parents found themselves in an unexpected position dealing with unfamiliar issues. Parents had to make sense of the unfamiliar and the information available to them was that gained from professionals or from media presentations of deafness (see Gregory 1991*a* for a discussion of this issue with respect to the role of the professional). Voysey (1975), in her study of families with disabled children, pointed out that families in different situations have to reflect upon their circumstances. 'Again if parents are to appear to be coping adequately with, and caring for the child, they must be able to present an orderly definition of his (sic) behaviour to others.'

The interview itself is, of course, a particular situation with particular rules and constraints. This does not invalidate it, but accounts given must be considered in this context. We were made aware in a number of ways that the interviewees were conscious of themselves in this role. We often felt that they had prepared themselves, sometimes taking up particular positions in the room, almost as if it were a theatre set. Often the behaviour prior to and after the interview was of a qualitatively different kind to that during the interview itself. There were changes in the style of talking or signing, and even in posture.

A number of parents told us that they had anticipated the interview with some trepidation, and for some it had meant reflecting on issues they usually chose not to think about.

> *When your letter came...If thoughts have come to mind in the past I've never wanted to get involved in talking about it. Maybe because my job is more than full-time, maybe because I don't want to think about it. If you'd said it did not matter whether you saw me or not I'd probably have said not.*

Perhaps we should reiterate here that there was no pressure for anyone to see us, although in our initial letter and first contact we did emphasise the importance to us of interviewing as many people as possible from the previous study. Most parents seemed to enjoy the experience of being interviewed.

> *Thank you for being so interested and for giving up a whole evening to talk to me.*

Parents of deaf sons and daughters and deaf young people themselves are groups whose views are seldom considered and some saw the interview as an opportunity to give us their perspective on various issues. Many felt that their unique experience made their comments particularly important, although their opinions had rarely been sought. Often it was clear that they had decided to use the interview to tell about specific concerns. This was particularly so with the later parent interview. They had already been interviewed once and most of them knew that a book had been published about their experience. As this interview was prearranged, they had time to prepare for it. It often emerged during the course of the interview that they had decided before we arrived to tell us particular things.

What was I going to tell you about that?

I was going to tell you...

And in some instances comments within the interview were clearly made for our benefit.

I honestly think looking back – I am saying this for you as much as for us – the more you can face up to what they have done and suffer the consequences to a certain extent, I am sure that is the better way.

In developing accounts, however, certain details could also be omitted, so the picture that emerged was one that the interviewee selected for the interview in terms of its purpose as they perceived it. Occasionally we were aware of deliberate omissions, and these often related to difficult periods in the life of the family. This, of course, is a legitimate choice for an interviewee to make. Where the young person had had an abortion, we were much more likely to learn this from the young woman herself than from the parents.

Occasionally, we were told information outside the interview that the parents did not want included as one of their responses. A prime example was in one of the interviews for the first book, when the mother asked for the tape recorder to be switched off. She then told sad and disturbing stories about the relationship between her young son and his father. Once it was switched on again she gave very neutral, ambiguous answers to a set of questions on the father-son involvement, attributing the poor relationship to the lack of time the father spent at home. We accept this as part of the research procedure and take the response of the interview as the account. There was only one instance where we felt we were being deliberately lied to, although even then we were not clear whether the young person was actually trying to deceive us, or engaging in her usual practice of telling elaborate stories for effect. Because the allegations she made about practices at her school were of such a serious nature, we made some further enquiries, which satisfied us that there was no foundation to them.

This does not imply that the interviews were a carefully prepared fabrication designed to impress or mislead us. Usually parents and young people wanted to give the most appropriate account they could of what had happened to them. They wanted other people and those they perceived to be in authority to understand their situation. They conveyed, in their attitude to us, that they did not see us as prying or as trying to obtain information from them that they did not want to reveal, but rather that we were in the position to let it be known how it really was.

Although some responses within the interview had clearly been rehearsed and others represented respondents' already established views on familiar issues, there were occasions when the interviewee seemed to be developing and articulating a previously undeveloped insight. Sometimes the parents and young people would construct their view of a particular topic as the interview progressed.

I wonder what I really think about that?

Well, I never knew I thought that.

Often a parent or young person expressed competing and logically contradictory views on a particular issue, both of which emerged during the process of the interview. Such inconsistencies in the views expressed often came about because the participant's views were not clearly developed on that topic or they were ambivalent on that issue. As was apparent in Chapter 2, for the parents, this often applied particularly to their views on communication which may have changed dramatically over time. Also, mothers and fathers could have different perspectives on the same topic, sometimes leading to disagreement between the two parents. Frequently, such contradictions were an indication of the various contexts in which people have to view their children. For example, in terms of the social comfort and ease of the deaf young person, one approach to education may seem best; in terms of academic attainment, it may be another.

Moreover, because we interviewed the parents twice and young people once, often covering the same topics in the interviews, we could see differences in their perspectives. Variations between parents and young people were seen in such issues as friendship and attendance at Deaf Club. Variations in parents' attitudes were seen, for example, in changing accounts of the cause of deafness. It is easy to explain these in terms of a changing understanding of differing perspectives. All of these accounts had their own validity, and certainly ambiguities and anomalies are not an indication of deliberate deception or untenable positions. We were certainly not aware of deliberate attempts to mislead us or to paint artificially rosy pictures, or gloomy ones.

In offering answers to questions, the young people and parents made sense of their experience in the most appropriate way they could, relative to the question. In writing this book we too have been engaged in a similar process. We have made the best sense of the information we have in the best way we could. As the interviewees offered different constructions of their experience, we offer different constructions of our evidence to give a range of complementary accounts.

At times this has meant constraining responses by placing them into coding categories in order to obtain an overview, and at other times we have explored in detail the actual way in which comments were made. Coding severely limits the responses by imposing categories that fit to varying degrees. Sometimes contradictions in the interviews presented problems in coding and in all cases we tried to be as faithful to the family as possible. It is, of course, an artificial activity, for while making data easier to handle and present, it introduces a simplicity that can fail to adequately show the complexity of peoples' lives. Yet this procedure opens up possibilities in other directions by allowing links to be made and relationships indicated.

We have been interested to see the issues that have received definite and unvarying treatment by respondents and those where the opinions held are clearly ambivalent, or where views are at variance with each other. We have tried in our discussion in the book to indicate the nature of the evidence we are considering on each particular topic. As far as possible our quantitative results are illustrated by quotes and elaborated discussion to allow the reader to judge their appropriateness. We hope the reader will find that the various accounts add to, rather than detract from, the total picture, by allowing exploration of the complex issues involved.

CONSTRUCTING THE INTERVIEW SCHEDULE

Constructing an interview that enables people to account for their experience in a way that is valid for them is not simple. In the early stages of the research we held a number of discussions with a range of people to identify relevant issues. Both our interview schedules were then piloted a number of times. However, in this research there were additional concerns. Firstly, the way in which the questions were constructed was likely in itself to presuppose a particular model or view of deafness. With such a topic, where the attitudes of the general population are usually negative and based on a deficiency model, we were concerned that the questions should not endorse such a view. In analysing the Office of Population Censuses and Surveys (OPCS) survey (published by Harris, 1971) Oliver points to the bias in the questions they asked by suggesting alternatives.

Does your health/disability affect your work in any way at present?

could be

Do you have problems at work because of the physical environment or the attitude of others? Oliver, 1990

However, to achieve this is more difficult than it might at first seem. A question such as, 'Would life be different if you were not deaf?' was seen by some as incorporating a negative evaluation of deafness. Yet the similar question, 'Would life be different if you were not red-haired?' or 'not clever?' would not elicit the same criticisms. The negative evaluation was in fact consequent upon the already pre-existing or presumed attitudes to deafness. In the parents' interview we tried to counteract this by highlighting the problem, by asking unanticipated questions, and by allowing the parents an opportunity to comment on the schedule itself.

With the young people this was more difficult. Because we wanted to explore the use of our interviews with the young people in some detail, after the research had been completed we held a meeting of notetakers who had been present at the interviews to comment on their experience of the validity and appropriateness of the interview. Eight notetakers attended, who had been present at 46 (75%) of the young people interviews. The ideas from this meeting inform some of the discussion here. Many of the notetakers saw the interview as negative, with too much emphasis on problems. Many reported that they came away from the interviews feeling depressed. We ourselves are not convinced that we did have an unduly heavy emphasis on problems; it may have been a reflection of the young people's experiences. We do accept, though, that beginning the interview with a number of questions focusing on hearing loss may have introduced the wrong emphasis, particularly in view of our rejection of hearing loss as a way of categorising the young people. However, not to do so would also have been problematic, as the rationale for interviewing was the young person's deafness.

Questions on family relationships did tend to ask the young people to reflect upon problems. However, an attempt to introduce a contrasting view often led to confusion or misunderstanding. A question such as, 'Do you think life has been any better for your family because you are deaf?' tended to be disorientating in the interview rather than giving interviewees an opportunity to evaluate deafness in a more positive way. However, the set of questions on feelings about being deaf towards the end of the interview did elicit responses highlighting the wider social context of the interviewees' situation and offering a range of responses, many of which challenged generally held views about deafness in society.

A further complexity in constructing the interview with the young people was the different languages and modes of presentation that needed to be used. With young people the interview could be presented in English (either orally or using SSE) or through BSL or using a combination sometimes including natural gesture.

For convenience, the young people's interview was initially developed in English. We created a written form that evolved on the basis of discussion with others and ideas that arose in the piloting stage. This meant that when the interview was conducted in BSL, it was always a translation from English. This may have been an error on our part. We believed at the time, and our experiences in interviewing confirmed this, that virtually all the young deaf people would have been introduced to English as their first language even if their preferred language at the time of the interview was BSL. This seemed to justify evolving the interview in English first. However, we accept that this may have disadvantaged BSL users in some respects, both in the structure of the interview as a whole and in the structure of individual questions. Systematic modifications were made for BSL interviews. The questions on the attitude scale were changed from direct statements for comment to a choice question, e.g. Margaret Thatcher is a good Prime Minister became MARGARET THATCHER, PRIME MINISTER, GOOD BAD, WHICH?

This may not be adequate, although we would ask our critics to consider the difficulties involved. Is it possible to develop two schedules in different languages in parallel? Even if this happened there would be difficulties in presentation, as the interview often switched between the two languages. Two different interviews may also have been criticised because of the potential for bias.

UNDERSTANDING QUESTIONS AND UNDERSTANDING ANSWERS

An issue in interviewing the deaf young people was whether or not they understood the questions and the extent to which we could make sense of some of the answers they gave. In Chapter 1 we comment on the number that could not be interviewed because of poor language skills (eight) and the number for whom, although the interview was carried out, levels of incomprehension or misunderstanding were so great that the results had to be excluded from the quantitative analysis (six). These exclusions affect the representative nature of the results presented in this study. In addition, throughout the book, for every question where responses are reported, we indicate the proportion that could not be included, because of difficulties in comprehension. This varied from 0 to 48% depending on the individual question, and for many issues was a substantial proportion. This further diminished the extent to which the findings could be said to be representative of the particular group of young people.

As one would expect, the most straightforward questions were answered by the greatest number. All (to whom the question applied) could answer the following.

Are you happy in this job? (applied to 43/61)

Do you read a newspaper?

Do you watch television?

The list of questions that could not be coded for over one-third of the group will illustrate where the difficulties lay.

Do you feel your school expected too much of you? (48%)

Were you treated differently by your parents because you were deaf? (44%)

Now I am going to ask you a 'just suppose' question. If you had a deaf child/teenager coming up to leaving school would you encourage him or her to get some experience of working? (43%)

Do you know why you are deaf? (38%)

When you were at school what technical aids did you use? (35%)

Do you think speaking deaf people are cleverer than signing deaf people? 34%

Very rarely was the problem simply one of language use, although one or two terms presented problems. More often, the difficulty was conceptual, in that deaf young people were asked to reflect upon how things might have been different or what they themselves would do in hypothetical situations.

Notetakers reported that the concepts that were difficult included 'technical aids' and 'voluntary work'. Some terms that were understood at the superficial level were difficult in respect of their implications within the specific questions, because the context was not understood. 'Is there anything about yourself you do not like and want to change?' was sometimes interpreted as being specific about changing clothes or hairstyle rather than more general issues. Some young people gave specific responses to questions where general ones were anticipated. A question about breakdown in parents' marriage, 'How did you feel when they split up?', could lead to responses about events at the actual time when one partner had left the family home. The most difficult questions were considerations of hypothetical situations.

If you had a deaf child...

Would life have been different...?

In addition, difficulty in communication meant that a number of deaf young people had developed specific strategies to cope with interaction, either nodding or smiling or agreeing with everything said or building answers around one or two specific words or signs that were used in the question. 'What kind of a person are you ?' could result in the answer, 'Yes I am a kind person'.

In raising these points we do not want to suggest in any way that it is not possible to ask such questions of deaf people, or that deaf people are unable to reflect upon these concerns. From our own experience, both within the interview situation and beyond, we know that discussion of these topics is not the prerogative of hearing people and that deaf people consider and reflect upon these themes. The concern is the poor language skills of some of the deaf young people, their development of communication strategies that are counter-productive to full communication, the unfamiliarity with particular concepts and ways of thinking, and the lack of experience of being asked about their own feelings, attitudes and desires. We regret that some of the deaf young people remain under-represented. Our concern in this appendix is the implications for such interview studies with young deaf people that any study in this area has to address.

We hope that in presenting these concerns as directly, honestly and frankly as we are able, we will not lessen the impact of the research, but further illustrate the issues involved. We ourselves do not see this as undermining the results presented but as a significant finding of the research itself.

INDEX